Sheelagh

here's to
greater health,

happiness

+

# Energy Now!

Michele
Cederberg

# Energy Now!

## SMALL STEPS
## TO AN ENERGETIC LIFE

Michelle Cederberg, MKin, BA, CEP

First Sentient Publications edition 2012
Copyright © 2012 by Michelle Cederberg

A paperback original

Cover and book design by Kim Johansen, Black Dog Design, www.blackdogdesign.com

Library of Congress Cataloging-in-Publication Data

Cederberg, Michelle, 1969-
  Energy now! : small steps to an energetic life / Michelle Cederberg. --
1st Sentient Publications ed.
      p. cm.
  1. Self-care, Health--Popular works. 2. Vitality--Popular works. 3.
Fatigue--Prevention--Popular works. I. Title.
  RA776.95.C43 2012
  613--dc23
                                    2011047395

Printed in the United States

10 9 8 7 6 5 4 3 2 1

SENTIENT PUBLICATIONS
A Limited Liability Company
1113 Spruce Street
Boulder, CO 80302
www.sentientpublications.com

For Ewan and Lilly

My daily source of love, support, and of course, energy.

# CONTENTS

FOREWORD ........................................................................... 11

PREFACE .............................................................................. 13

ACKNOWLEDGEMENTS ............................................................ 15

**INTRODUCTION.** NOT ANOTHER BOOK
ON PERSONAL HEALTH? ........................................................ **17**

Your Energy Now! Reader's Guide ...................................... 18

Decide and Conquer .......................................................... 20

Assess Your Energy Now ................................................... 21

NEED ENERGY? ............................................................... 21

How Did You Rate? ........................................................... 23

**PART 1. MAKE UP YOUR MIND** **25**

**CHAPTER 1.** FROM TIRED, WIRED, AND READY TO DROP
TO ENERGY NOW! ................................................................ **27**

Dropping the Ball .............................................................. 31

I Blew It ............................................................................ 32

Baby, Come Back! .............................................................. 32

CHARGE! ......................................................................... 33

Whatever It Takes (*Darren's Story*) .................................... 35

ENERGY NOW! First Steps ................................................. 36

**CHAPTER 2.** THE ENERGY NOW! PHILOSOPHY ........................... **39**

Get Your Body Out of Debt ................................................ 40

All in Good Time ............................................................... 41

Look After the Pennies and the Pounds Look After Themselves .............. 42

Four Arguments against *Going Big* ..................................... 43

Dream BIG but Start Small ................................................................ 48

CHARGE! ........................................................................................ 49

Whatever It Takes (*Small Steps Quantified*) .............................. 51

ENERGY NOW! Small Steps with Food and Fitness ........................ 53

**CHAPTER 3. THE TEN ENERGY COMMANDMENTS** .......................... **55**

Whatever It Takes (*My Reality Check*) ...................................... 62

CHARGE! Write your personal growth mantra .................................. 64

ENERGY NOW! 10 Energy Commandments ................................ 65

**CHAPTER 4. TAKING DOWN THE TIME BANDITS** ........................... **67**

It's a Matter of Priority .................................................................. 67

Look at the Time! ............................................................................ 68

Prioritizing You ............................................................................ 69

Small Steps to Great Gains! .......................................................... 75

CHARGE! ........................................................................................ 77

Whatever It Takes (*Learn to Say No*) ........................................ 78

ENERGY NOW! Schedule in YOU ................................................ 79

**PART 2. TAKE CARE OF YOUR BODY** **81**

**CHAPTER 5. FITNESS: EXERCISE LESS FOR SUCCESS** ...................... **83**

Finally Fitting in Fitness ................................................................ 86

Four Steps to Exercise Success .................................................... 87

Happy Heart .................................................................................... 92

Mighty Muscles .............................................................................. 94

Stay Real ........................................................................................ 96

CHARGE! ........................................................................................ 97

Whatever It Takes (*Jackie's Story*) ............................................ 97

ENERGY NOW! Exercise Less ...................................................... 98

**CHAPTER 6. NUTRITION: FUELLING A NEW YOU ONE BITE**

**AT A TIME** .................................................................................... **101**

Bite-sized Nutrition Changes You Can Swallow ............................ 103

Back to Basics ................................................................................ 104

Energize Your Eating .................................................................... 112

Size Matters! .................................................................................. 117

CHARGE!......................................................................... 122

Whatever It Takes (*Valerie's Story*) ................................ 123

ENERGY NOW! Nourishing Nibbles.............................. 125

**CHAPTER 7.** HYDRATION: *Water You Drinking?* ........................... **127**

Water *Works* ................................................................... 128

Exercise and Fluid Replacement ...................................... 133

Checks and Balances........................................................ 134

Less Sodas, Juices, and Sugary Drinks ............................. 135

CHARGE!......................................................................... 137

Whatever It Takes ........................................................... 137

ENERGY NOW! Make Hydration a Habit ...................... 138

**CHAPTER 8.** SLEEP: THE QUEST FOR REST AND RELAXATION.......... **141**

Zzzzzzz's PLEASE! ........................................................... 142

Benefits of Sleep ............................................................. 143

How Much Is Enough? .................................................... 145

Sleep Routine ................................................................. 146

Sleep Environment ......................................................... 149

CHARGE!......................................................................... 154

Whatever It Takes ........................................................... 154

Energy NOW! Sleep Tight ............................................... 155

**CHAPTER 9.** STRESS LESS FOR SUCCESS........................................... **157**

Stress Express.................................................................. 158

Chronic Stress, Energy and Creativity ............................. 160

Stress Awareness ............................................................. 161

Stress Defense ................................................................. 163

CHARGE!......................................................................... 168

Whatever It Takes ........................................................... 169

ENERGY NOW! Stress Stoppers....................................... 170

**PART 3. FEED YOUR SPIRIT**      **173**

**CHAPTER 10.** THE HAPPINESS FACTOR ......................................... **175**

The Leaky Toilet Test ..................................................... 176

Positive Identification .................................................... 178

CHARGE!......................................................................... 183

Whatever It Takes (*Unhappy Me*) ............................................................ 183
ENERGY NOW! The Happiness Factor ............................................ 184

**CHAPTER 11.** THE KINDNESS EXPERIMENT .................................. **187**
People Power .............................................................................................. 188
CHARGE! ..................................................................................................... 194
Whatever It Takes (*Positive Tickets*) .......................................................... 195
ENERGY NOW! Please Be Kind ................................................................ 195

**CHAPTER 12.** THE PASSION PROJECT ............................................. **197**
The Energy Connection ......................................................................... 199
Find Your Own Everest ............................................................................ 200
Six Steps to Finding Your Own Everest .................................................... 201
CHARGE! ..................................................................................................... 209
Whatever It Takes .................................................................................... 210
ENERGY NOW! Recharge Your Passions ................................................. 211

**CHAPTER 13.** SMALL STEPS TO AN ENERGETIC LIFE ...................... **213**
Believe You Can Achieve Your Plan .......................................................... 214
CHARGE! ..................................................................................................... 226
Whatever It Takes .................................................................................... 226
ENERGY NOW! Stay on Track .................................................................. 227

REFERENCES ............................................................................................... 229
ABOUT THE AUTHOR ................................................................................. 237

# FOREWORD

**M**ICHELLE CEDERBERG's *Energy Now* is a genuine must-have in what is a congested genre, as she herself points out. My first glance down the contents pages and deeper into the structure of the book piqued my interest and also filled me with a sense of trepidation! Sure enough, as I read each chapter I thought "terrific stuff" and at the same time, "Wow, this is me...and many people I know!" So, suitably scolded, I paid increasing attention to the CHARGE!, Whatever It Takes, and Energy Now! elements and suggestions and found myself becoming equipped with a personalized action plan to bring myself (and my life) back under self control.

In essence, Michelle identifies quickly the critical areas where challenges arise. Then with clear messaging and practical guidance, she lays out a guiding framework for anyone who wishes to make positive changes to their life. One of the most important elements that distinguishes Michelle's advice and suggestions from the myriad of works in the area is the scope for individualization of a plan and action for change, rather than enforcing some antiseptic, only-one-way-to-do-things model. She manages this feat by providing a book packed with information, anecdotes, observations, and a wealth of relevant material from her experience and drive for self-learning. In other words, a two-dimensional written document that can greatly uplift a person's multi-dimensional life! *Thoroughly recommended*...and where did I put my To Do list? I need to make some (slight) alterations!

Stephen R. Norris, Ph.D.
Vice President, Sport, WinSport Canada

# PREFACE

ENERGY! If you've got lots of it you're laughing, but if you don't you know how difficult it is to generate. It's a paradox for the working tired: if you're low on energy you need to expend energy to get energy. How can you do that if you have no energy? Really good question.

I guess it's because so many of us struggle to find and keep good health and endless energy that everyone and his dog have a theory for how you can get it faster and with less effort. Quick fix? I say buyer beware!

Your healthy living plan should not be viewed as a race but as an ongoing, lifelong and even enjoyable journey. It isn't always easy… but I will tell you that it is possible. So here we go.

Through more than two decades as a motivational speaker, personal trainer, life coach, author and health educator I've observed a lot about human nature and our health practices. Here's what I know today.

The lack of energy you're experiencing right now is less about not knowing what to do and more about not knowing how to do it. You could get buried beneath the available books and resources that will tell you exactly what to do. You've got the information. Am I right?

The challenge you're facing as far as I can see it is how to get started and stay with it when the busy-life meter is at eleven and the energy gauge is at zero. Yup, the energy paradox: *If you're low on energy, you need to expend energy to get energy, and you have no energy.* To overcome this annoying dilemma you'll need a different approach.

I'm sure you're not new to the idea of small steps. A lot of self-help professionals support the idea in theory, but few create an entire methodology around it. It's not sexy enough. It won't bring results quickly enough.

But neither will sitting on the sofa, and that's likely where you end up every time your busy life closes in on another of the sexy, results-promising, go-big-or-go-home methods you've tried. And oh how you've tried.

There's no lack of desire is there? So if you had a way to gain better health, greater happiness and more energy that was compatible with your low-energy, busy life you'd be all over that wouldn't you?

Well here it is: an entire health and energy-generating methodology based on small, unsexy steps.

I wrote this book for you, open-minded and hopeful as you are. Just know this: the ultimate energetic life won't happen through physical means alone. In this book you'll gain insight into how mind, body and spirit all play in to your balanced energy plan.

Physical health and wellness are addressed for certain. Your strong, healthy body is the foundation on which you will build the happy, energetic life you crave.

We'll explore the power of the mind by looking at the mindset you carry about your own capabilities. *I can't do this, it's never worked, I'm not motivated, I'll start tomorrow.* If you allow negativity, self-doubt, and procrastination to rent space in your head, you've essentially made up your mind that you don't deserve a happy, healthy, energetic life. Let's get over that kind of thinking shall we?

And of course this book will help you understand that a life filled with more happiness, daily acts of kindness and projects and people you're passionate about is a life filled with limitless and inspiring energy. *Mind. Body. Spirit.* Excellent!

Small steps to an energetic life. Believe it. Harness a bit of the self-discipline you know you possess and decide that this time will be different.

I know you can. Let's figure it out together – one small step at a time, one page at a time, because that's all it takes.

# Acknowledgements

IT TAKES A LOT OF ENERGY TO WRITE A BOOK ABOUT ENERGY AND THIS one would not have happened without these very important people. My #1 thank you goes to Susan Sweeney, who selflessly gave her time and vast knowledge to coach me, Stephanie Staples and Lea Brovedani to write a book proposal, set a schedule and *actually* write the book instead of talking about it. Susan, without you I'd still be talking about it. And to Stephanie and Lea, my partners in productivity – this goal was way more fun to reach sharing it with the two of you. You three women rock!

I'm grateful to my publisher, Connie Shaw, for reading my proposal and making the call. Thank you for believing in me and this book. You're a pleasure to work with.

My assistant, Sarada Eastham, worked endlessly to compile and format my references and resources. Her efforts freed me up to focus on writing. She was also a real cheerleader as my deadlines loomed closer. A more positive person you will not meet.

As I wrote this book two heart beats played the central role in its completion. My sage and silly dog, Lilly, sat at my feet as I toiled, and helped me stretch my legs when I needed energy. What comfort. And the love of my life, Ewan Nicholson, sat by my side. Your insightful, sometimes brutal feedback made this a stronger book; your endless support and encouragement made this a tolerable process; and your love for me makes this a better life. Thank you all.

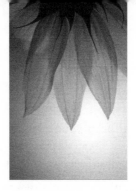

# INTRODUCTION

# Not Another Book on Personal Health?

## *Why You Need Energy Now!*

> *If I'd known I was going to live so long,*
> *I'd have taken better care of myself.*
> —LEON ELDRED ON HIS 104TH BIRTHDAY

S ERIOUSLY! *If one more perky, self-righteous, fitness freak tells me I can transform my life in twenty-one days by exercising seven days a week and simply cutting out bread, beer and anything that tastes good, I'm going to roll off the sofa and throw my doughnut at them!*

Annoying isn't it? Even if it's something you want or need, lifestyle change can be difficult – especially when the guidance is coming from someone who is already there and their methods require a painful overhaul of your entire life. *How could they possibly know how hard it is? They eat, sleep and breathe this stuff.*

When it comes to investing in your health and self-care you definitely have a lot of choices at your fingertips – too many in fact. The puzzling profusion of TV programs, DVDs, home equipment, online plans, endless books and over-the-top magazines selling the latest, greatest, fastest, best results will cause even the savvy shopper to surrender. If this has been your experience then I'm glad we found each other. But before we begin let me make one thing abundantly clear. Energy Now! *is not* a jumper-cable jolt back to life. While I'm sure a quick-fix energy solution would be convenient for your time strapped schedule, it's not what I'm about. If that's what you're after, you may as well give my book to the next person you see and keep looking because I won't be able to help you.

Energy Now! *won't* provide an instantaneous eraser for years of bad habits. Honestly, what possibly could? It can't deliver more energy, better health, and a recharged life tomorrow...but it can guide you on a realistic path to *start* right now – sapped of time and stamina though you may be.

You will get *energy* soon, and the best time to begin is *now*.

I know what you're thinking. *If I don't have any time, stamina, or motivation NOW to do what it takes to feel better, how is this going to work?* Great question! That's where my methods differ from the *17-secrets-to-change-your-life-in-30-seconds* philosophies that the media bombard us with. The Energy Now! approach helps you get energy *now* through small daily steps.

Everything you do, everything you want to accomplish can be broken down into smaller units that will fit in to your busy life.

Whether you are an in-demand executive, a multi-tasking mom, or an industrious entrepreneur – *heck, if you're retired, tired, or uninspired* – Energy Now! will provide you with small-steps advice to prioritize the energy-creating self-care practices you didn't think you had time for. Health, happiness and an energetic life are yours for the taking, starting now.

## YOUR ENERGY NOW! READER'S GUIDE

*Energy Now!* is divided into three sections, each with the goal to guide you mind, body and spirit on your path to a more energetic life.

The first section is called *Make Up Your Mind* and includes the first four chapters. This section will give you clarity about your change process, help you truly commit to your plan, and show you how to find time for yourself in a busy schedule.

Section 2, entitled *Take Care of Your Body*, encompasses five chapters that focus entirely on improving your physical health and wellness through exercise, nutrition, hydration, sleep and stress management. You'll gain a lot of very practical, fact-based information in these chapters along with my advice and tips for staying on track with your health no matter what.

The final section, called *Feed Your Spirit,* will do just that. When it comes to personal energy you probably think about physical health as the main way to get more of it. In truth your energy is created and lost in so many different ways beyond simple physical health. This section shows you the importance of emotional health on your personal energy through a closer look at happiness, kindness and passion.

At the end of this chapter you'll have the opportunity to complete an *energy quiz* that will help you identify your biggest energy drains. You likely already know what they are, but maybe you'll uncover a few surprises. Awareness strengthens change.

As you read through the chapters you'll notice four regular features, each with a goal to provide you with support and motivation, ideas and, of course, action steps.

## CHARGE!

At the end of each chapter I ask you to take action with some aspect of what you've just read. CHARGE! is meant to invoke the idea of taking charge of your situation, charging forward in attack, or charging your batteries – all of which have energy at their core and promote your progress.

I'll often ask you to write down your thoughts or goals around some topic, so have a pen handy. The requests will rarely require more than a few minutes of your time, and the very act of writing versus simply thinking about your answer will increase the chances that your thoughts will turn into actions.

## Whatever It Takes

Sometimes motivation comes to us from odd and interesting sources. Whatever It Takes shares success stories that promote self-discipline and motivation. I hope these segments will inspire you to do *whatever it takes* to accomplish your goals.

## Energy Now!

Better energy comes to you from so many sources in your life. Not just through eating right and exercise. At the end of each chapter you will find a fast glance *Energy Now!* list full of simple, quick ideas related to what you've just read in that chapter. Even if all you do is execute a few of these energy-producing habits every day, your lethargy will leave you and your get-up-and-go will put on a show. Hmmmm, that might be worth a bit of your effort don't you think?

## Free Dose of Energy Now

Throughout the book you'll notice sidebars that send you to my website where you can gather extra resources, tips and exercises to expand your Energy Now! experience. Take the time to visit the site every time you get a new access word, and up your dose of energy now.

# DECIDE AND CONQUER

So here we go. You've made the decision to take charge of your health, energy and happiness, and I want you to experience success.

From this point forward ignore your inner critic. Shut down the little voice that tells you *I can't do it, it hasn't worked before, I'm too lazy, I'm unmotivated, I'm too tired...* That voice is operating on old assumptions and is leading you astray.

Decide today that change is possible for you, and allow the information in this book to guide you on a new path to success. Say it with me now: *I can do this. I will remain open-minded. I am strong, motivated and capable!*

Do it just because you can. This book will show you how.

## Assess Your Energy Now

You're probably in the market for an energy boost or two, or you wouldn't have picked up this book. Well I'm glad you did because I know my methods can help you find what you're looking for. Before you read on, take a moment to complete my *Energy Now! Assessment*. It will only take moments and will no doubt increase your awareness of all the ways you gain and drain energy every day. It will also remind you of what you're already doing right in your quest for more energy. Complete the assessment as a starting point for your success.

### The Energy Now! Assessment

## 🖱 FREE DOSE OF ENERGY NOW

To complete your Energy Now! Assessment online
go to *www.worklifeenergy.com*, register if you are a
first time user, and enter ENERGY in the E-NOW box.

## NEED ENERGY?

Your lifestyle behaviors can have a big impact on your day-to-day energy levels. Take my twenty-questions Energy Now! quiz to note your potential energy drains. Read the questions below and check the answer that corresponds with your current state.

## ENERGY NOW ASSESSMENT

| RATE YOURSELF on each of the questions below by checking the appropriate box. | YES (I got it going on) | SOMETIMES (I'm hit and miss) | NO (I'm stuck at STOP) |
|---|---|---|---|
| **MAKE UP YOUR MIND** | | | |
| 1) I have enough energy to get through my day | ☐ | ☐ | ☐ |
| 2) I'm generally happy and I like my life | ☐ | ☐ | ☐ |
| 3) I regularly find time for myself | ☐ | ☐ | ☐ |
| 4) I have someone I can talk to when I need to | ☐ | ☐ | ☐ |
| 5) I rarely worry | ☐ | ☐ | ☐ |
| 6) I get tasks done in a timely manner | ☐ | ☐ | ☐ |
| **TAKE CARE OF YOUR BODY** | | | |
| 7) I feel good about my current level of physical health | ☐ | ☐ | ☐ |
| 8) I exercise at least three times each week | ☐ | ☐ | ☐ |
| 9) I drink enough hydrating fluids each day | ☐ | ☐ | ☐ |
| 10) I am happy and realistic about my eating habits | ☐ | ☐ | ☐ |
| 11) I generally make good food choices through the day | ☐ | ☐ | ☐ |
| 12) I avoid skipping meals throughout the day | ☐ | ☐ | ☐ |
| 13) I regularly get enough sleep | ☐ | ☐ | ☐ |
| 14) I am a non-smoker and avoid secondhand smoke | ☐ | ☐ | ☐ |

**FEED YOUR SPIRIT**

| | | | |
|---|---|---|---|
| 15) I generally manage my stress well | ☐ | ☐ | ☐ |
| 16) I get satisfaction from my career or chosen path | ☐ | ☐ | ☐ |
| 17) I have hobbies I enjoy and engage in regularly | ☐ | ☐ | ☐ |
| 18) I laugh daily | ☐ | ☐ | ☐ |
| 19) I regularly find time for my family and friends | ☐ | ☐ | ☐ |
| 20) I am responsible with my spending | ☐ | ☐ | ☐ |

# How Did You Rate?

STUCK AT STOP? If you answered *no* to most questions it's time for a serious *energy injection* in your life! The good news is you now have a better idea of what you need to work on, and you've started on the path to a healthier, more energetic life. Work to improve one or two habits at a time.

HIT AND MISS? If you're on-again-off-again with your habits, *pay attention – something is about to change.* If you answered *sometimes* to a lot of these questions, it's either because you're improving yourself and heading for YES or because you're falling off the wagon and headed for oh NO! Your goal is to create more consistency with your hit and miss habits so they shift to GO. *I've got ideas that can help!*

YES EXPRESS! If you've "got it going on" with most of your responses you should be proud of yourself! Don't rest on your laurels though. Take a look at any hit and miss or oh NO responses and give them a bit of attention. Give yourself a pat on the back and keep up the good work.

# PART 1

## Make Up Your Mind

YOU'VE GOT A DECISION TO MAKE. You picked up this book because you want something in your life to change or improve, right? How many times have you tried before this?

If you've come up against barriers in previous attempts to get healthy and energized you know that there is a little more to it than simply pressing go. Procrastination and avoidance still manage to rear their ugly heads even when you've set a goal you really want to achieve. What's up with that?

This is why, in my version of mind, body and spirit the mind part is all about making up your mind that you want change and deserve it. In the next three chapters I want you to become mindful of what needs to be in place so you can get a good start and stay on track no matter how crazy life gets.

I want you to remind yourself what you need to do better or differently this time so you can be assured of a successful outcome.

I want you to gain clarity about your change process – the challenges and triumphs you'll face, the good and the bad that will arise – so you can truly commit to a new and energetic life once and for all. No surprises.

Make up your mind and then lay the foundation for success. Decide and conquer, baby! This time things are going to be different.

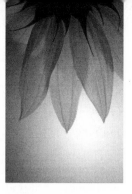

CHAPTER 1

# From Tired, Wired, and Ready to Drop to Energy NOW!

---

*The bad news is time flies. The good news is you're the pilot.*
—MICHAEL ALTSHULER

---

I MAGINE *your perfect energy-filled day.* You wake up before your alarm and feel refreshed and excited about the day that lies ahead. You're up early enough that you don't need to rush out the door, so you make a proper breakfast and enjoy the morning with your family. As you glance at the newspaper headlines you make a plan to walk the dog before you leave for work and remind yourself to pack your lunch and a bag for the gym.

You have a noon workout scheduled with a friend. You're excited to get to the office so you can finish that proposal you've been working on and begin preparing the presentation that will help sell it. You love your job. You work hard at it but you also value time with family and friends so you created a schedule that allows for maximum productivity without the long hours. You get more done in four hours of work than most people do in a full day. It's amazing what you can get accomplished when you've got energy and clarity on your side.

You leave the office before rush hour and have time to spend with your kids before making a scrumptious dinner together with your partner. Since you don't have to bring your work home with you, the evening is about family, friends, fun, and relaxation. You've got your health, a sense of life balance, and energy to spare. Life is good. Actually, life is GREAT!

*HA! Are you #$%@in' kidding me?* You get up early only because you have to. You don't have time to eat breakfast. You commute to work in your car every day for *at least* thirty minutes in each direction and mainline coffee from morning until 2:00 p.m.

Around 9:00 a.m. you grab a doughy treat at the coffee place near your office. You sit at your desk for the better part of eight hours a day with the occasional stretch for the phone, or "anaerobic burst" for the elevator at quitting time. Lunch requires a trip down to the food court so you get a bit of exercise then but you don't have time to work out. You don't have the energy either.

By the time you get home you can't see straight for exhaustion so if you had a dog it would be overweight too. Your kids know not to bug you because you're usually tired and irritable or snoring on the sofa before dinner. If you *are* involved in activity with them it's typically sitting at the side of the soccer field or dance class, watching them do their thing. You channel surf for a few hours after dinner, scramble to get the last of the day's errands done and if you're lucky you fall into bed by 11:30 p.m. dog-tired, still wired, and wishing for a magical solution to get energy now.

As frustrating and depressing as it may sound, far more people identify with the second scenario over the first. We're tired, wired, and ready to drop. These days we're working more than ever, spending less time with our friends and family and inevitably watching our health and happiness drift away. We are far more familiar with stress, sleep deprivation, fast food and lack of exercise than we are with health, vitality and energy.

More than half of North Americans are sedentary – not exercising at levels high enough to maintain basic health. As a result, diseases of lifestyle like diabetes, heart disease, hypertension and obesity have risen to epidemic levels negatively affecting our wellbeing and depleting our already dwindling energy levels. To add insult to injury, sleep deprivation contributes to high levels of daytime drowsiness and lowered productivity on the job.

Are you one of the *working tired*? Too busy or fatigued to take care of yourself, you see the weight creep on and the energy move out, and before long you're dealing with poor fitness levels and health challenges of your own. Well, you're not alone. You are among millions of North Americans experiencing a real-life personal energy crisis – too much to do and not enough time, stamina or motivation to do it.

Busy people everywhere unite with the common exasperated admission: *I'm tired all the time!* The health and energy you possessed in your twenties has gradually been exhausted under the burden of long hours and increasing pressures at work plus added responsibilities and family commitments at home.

Somewhere along the way you took yourself off your own priority list and now suffer from some combination of poor health, high levels of fatigue and ever-present stress.

I once had a client just like this. Darren had always been driven. In university he got top grades, had good friends, was a first string varsity basketball player and had a passion for the outdoors. He valued hard work but also knew the benefits of staying in shape and having fun.

He landed a great job straight out of school and quickly found himself on the fast track to a good life. When he got married and had children, he was able to provide well for his family. It sometimes meant long hours but it was all for a good cause. They could afford a nice house and a new car and the kids were able to take part in all sorts of activities.

Darren spent less time doing the activities he loved but he told himself it was just temporary. He would work hard now to make and save money to pay down some debt and when things were less hectic he'd get back to the gym, spend more time with his friends and family and get back on track.

Pretty soon Darren was asked to become a partner in the business. What a great opportunity! His hard work had paid off and he and his family would reap the benefits.

It wasn't long before Darren was not only putting in longer work days but he was also working occasional weekends. He couldn't remember the last time he had exercised or done something fun with his kids. He had gained weight, was starting to feel fatigue and stress all the time and wondered if that pain in his chest was indigestion or something he should really worry about.

He no longer had energy and because of that he was unmotivated to do anything about it. It seemed that Darren's fast track to the good life had brought his health to a grinding halt.

When I first met Darren he was eighty pounds overweight, looked older than his years, got winded tying his shoes, and couldn't remember the last time he didn't feel tired. He came to me for personal training in a desperate bid to regain his health, get more energy and feel better about himself.

He suffered from high blood pressure, borderline diabetes and a whole host of other health challenges resulting from inactivity, poor diet and lousy self-care practices. A few weeks earlier his doctor had told him it was time to make some serious lifestyle changes or he wouldn't be around much longer. That news scared him because he was only thirty-eight years old.

Darren, like so many hardworking people today battled to balance the responsibilities of a growing career and family with the necessity of taking care of self. He stepped into action that day and began *his* journey of transformation. Darren's story may have different characters and circumstances, but perhaps you can relate?

Somewhere along the way you stopped taking care of yourself and your health and now you're sick and tired all the time. You've likely looked for ways to get motivated – health and fitness programs or DVDs, a new gym, a personal trainer who looks like you want to, television programs creating unrealistic expectations, the latest fitness gizmo or über-diet promising big results, internet sites spreading conflicting information, or maybe one of the endless magazines and books promoting the latest and greatest trend in regaining health and energy. The "help" choices are vast to the point of being overwhelming, but are they working?

Remember that the definition of *insanity* is doing the same thing over and over again and expecting different results. It's insane! If so many people are still inactive and unhealthy perhaps it's time for a different, simpler approach to get energized? If you drop the ball again, leave it where it is and pick up a different ball!

## DROPPING THE BALL

When your life gets busy and out of control, what are the first items that get dropped from your to-do list? Be honest. Essential tasks like your job, childcare and household duties can't be negotiated; that nap when you get home is the only way you'll survive until bed time; social time after work or TV time at night rarely gets skipped; and surfing the internet or playing that video game still seem to find their way into your busy day.

Yet in times of stress and fatigue most people are quick to give up important self-care priorities like exercise, healthy eating and getting enough sleep when the physical resilience they bring is the exact weapon you need against fatigue and stress. What's worse is that you'll tell yourself you don't have time for them either.

You fool yourself into believing productivity is more important than personal care. *Think of all I will get done if I just skip my workout!*

You give up sleep and fuel yourself on coffee and muffins to gain a few more hours to slay the never-ending to-do list.

You distract yourself from stress through harmful habits like smoking or excess alcohol consumption, often believing that the stress will be short lived and healthy habits will return in short order. *It won't always be this way. I just have to get through this busy time!* Before you know it, you've blown it.

# I BLEW IT

In my life as a personal trainer new clients would often come to me in a state of shock. They would look in the mirror one day and see a tired, overweight face staring back at them and wonder how it came to this.

Several years ago a client named Sarah admitted to me quite incredulously, *I didn't mean to get fat. I really don't know how it happened!* And she *really* didn't. Sarah never intended to let things get so far out of control. She confessed that she always had it in the back of her mind to make better choices and get back to exercising. She always intended to get out and walk or go to the gym and every now and again she would. She *always* thought about getting more sleep or eating better.

The small efforts here and there helped her feel like she was moving in the right direction but more often than not, intention surpassed action and the habits didn't stick. All the while she held steadfast to her belief that she would eventually create a habit around her health and as she so openly stated, *In the process of waiting for the big inspiration, I got FAT.*

So powerful are our intentions to do good for ourselves that it surprises us when our bodies don't keep up with the dialogue in our minds. *Overweight, out of shape, and tired... where did YOU come from?*

# BABY, COME BACK!

Over the years I've heard dozens of clients admit that getting *back* in shape required so much more effort than getting *out* of shape in the first place. Every last one of them wished they hadn't let their health go.

Maybe you're thinking the same thing. But hindsight is 20/20 and here you are with a decision to make about your health: keep looking back on all your mistakes, or find a way to focus forward for change. The choice to put yourself back on your priority list is an obvious one but it sure isn't easy. If it was, we wouldn't be in the middle of a North American health epidemic and you wouldn't need this book.

Yes, it's easy to become demoralized when everything feels like an effort and results don't come quickly enough. It's probably why so few penitent couch potatoes reach their objective the first time out of the gate…or even the second…or the seventh. *Sigh*… Those who experience success are the ones who simply decide *enough already! I'll do whatever it takes.*

I won't claim that the path to energy, health and a recharged life is easy, simple, or even always fun. I've been a health enthusiast for over twenty years and I *still* have days when I don't want to exercise. I have moments when I wish chicken wings were good for you and I often wish TV watching burned calories.

Exercise is tiring, healthy eating takes time, early-to-bed seems boring and – darn it anyway – french fries taste good! I get it, and we're going to talk about it, but first you have to make a commitment to get on board the energy train and see where this ride could take you.

Yes, it will require some effort on your part but not in the ways that you think. You'll have some tough days but you'll have more victorious ones.

So you're stepping outside your comfort zone. What if you decide to go for it anyway and through consistent, small steps you are able to feel great again? It might be a risk worth taking. And really, do you have any other choice?

## CHARGE!

Take charge of your health. It really doesn't matter how busy, stressed, and tired you are. If you live and breathe on this planet you have a responsibility to yourself *and* your loved ones to take care of yourself by whatever means possible.

There is a reason this book found its way to you, so what's it going to take? A little more weight around the mid-section? High blood pressure? Diabetes? A heart attack? If you're ignoring your health it's not a matter of *if* you'll be afflicted with one or more of the growing list of diseases of lifestyle it's *when*.

The good news is you can feel better again regardless of your current age, fitness level, or past experiences and you can begin right now.

1. If you haven't already done so, make sure you complete your *Energy Now! Assessment* at *www.worklifeenergy.com*. It will only take a moment and the information will increase your awareness on your path to change.

2. Look to the future and envision the new you. Healthy, vibrant, energized. Picture how you look, imagine how you feel, think of all the things you're able to do, and tell your *today* self what it's like. Keep that vision in mind as you complete these sentences:

The best thing about having more energy is:

I'm so happy because now I can:

I never thought I'd be able to do this, but I plan to:

Along your path to more energy, better health, and a recharged life remind yourself of the words you wrote above and use them to stay on course. You're on your way.

## Whatever It Takes (*Darren's Story*)

Remember Darren from the start of this chapter: a thirty-eight-year-old hard working, successful husband and father of two who had neglected his health and self-care? He was eighty pounds overweight, fatigued and stressed out, suffering from high blood pressure, borderline diabetes and a whole host of other health challenges.

He had no time and no energy, and had come to see me mostly because his doctor told him he should. He didn't want to be there and if he wasn't so scared that he would die too young he would have quit before he started. He told me so.

Darren needed structure and breadth to his health resurrection so we agreed on a weekly small-steps plan he would follow – no matter what.

Here's what it looked like.

- Every day Darren parked his car at a lot that was further from his office. It necessitated an eight-minute walk there and back every day. He often used this time to make a phone call, or just to collect his thoughts as he walked.
- Every week we scheduled two personal training sessions where I made him work as hard as he could handle.
- Every week Darren committed to doing one more exercise session on his own. It was usually a simple thirty- or forty-minute treadmill walk or stationary bike ride.
- Every week Darren chose two work days where he would leave precisely at quitting time so he could pick up his kids from school and spend some quality Dad time with them.
- On those two days he also committed to getting to bed earlier.
- Every week Darren made small nutrition improvements. Week one, he cut out sodas. Week two, he changed what he ate for breakfast. Grilled ham and three eggs with buttery toast became two poached eggs on dry toast and some fruit.
- Week three, he added in healthy snacks. Week four, he stopped eating potato chips in the evenings.

...and so on. Small changes. You should know that Darren continued to eat out for lunch meetings, often ordering large pasta meals or a burger and fries. He also maintained his post-work cold beer (or two). He told me he wanted *some* fun in his life! That was all right though because the small changes he committed to still amounted to worthwhile results.

That's where the list started. We added to it and changed things up as Darren began to see results. I'll be honest though, the changes came slowly at first and they weren't without their ups and downs. But they came.

In the first three months of his new plan Darren lost only nine pounds – the equivalent of about ¾ pound per week, but he definitely had more energy and noticed differences in how his clothes fit. He also saw improvements with his health. His blood pressure dropped and his cholesterol profile improved.

He kept at it and stepped up his exercise and healthy eating efforts. Six months into his new plan he was down almost twenty-five pounds and was no longer at risk for diabetes.

As Darren lost weight, his health problems improved and his confidence and energy soared. It took him about eighteen months to get close to his goal weight and he did it by starting with small steps that would be manageable even when his busy life wasn't.

No one says change has to happen in giant leaps in order to be effective. Darren embraced the *whatever it takes* mentality and look where it took him!

## ENERGY NOW!

### First Steps

The list below includes small efforts you can make *this week* to begin on your path to improved energy. Don't wait until you've finished reading the book. Pick one idea each day, or choose a few to implement through the week. Keep it simple. Just do it, and if it feels good, *keep doing it!*

- Replace at least one soda, juice, or sugary drink with a big glass of water.

- Set a timer to remind you to stand up and move around for five minutes every sixty minutes.

- Climb the stairs (at least two flights) instead of taking the elevator or escalator.

- Eat breakfast. Last night's pizza counts.

- Turn off the TV thirty minutes before bed (think of what else you could do before bed to relax and wind down).

- Schedule in time for yourself to do something fun.

- Clear the clutter in your bedroom. You'll sleep better.

- Breathe deeply – right to the bottom of your lungs – several times throughout the day.

- Get some fresh air on your coffee break. Smoke breaks don't count!

- Minimize coffee to two cups per day. Drink water the rest of the time.

- Ban the vending machine as a food source.

- Stretch tight muscles as you sit at your desk.

- Have another glass of water.

- When that sugar craving hits, eat fruit!

- Sit and stand with better posture.

- Take five minutes to write down ten things you love about yourself. Read it daily.

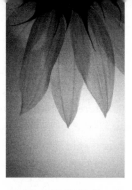

CHAPTER 2

# The Energy Now! Philosophy

*Confront the difficult while it is still easy; accomplish
the great task by a series of small acts.*
—Tao Te Ching

WHEN I present to audiences, one of the core messages I repeat again and again is the concept of *small steps toward great gains.* Anything worth doing is worth taking action on *now* even with a small step, rather than waiting for more time and the hope of a bigger, more ideal step down the road.

*Why do we have such a difficult time applying that theory to our own self-care?* I hear it all the time. *What's the point? Why would I bother with such a small effort when it won't help me?*

If you're among the masses who have been brain-washed with a *more is better* message that small efforts are wasted efforts, listen up. In the process of waiting for the heavens to open and shower you with the abundance of time and motivation you *think* you need, you're wasting valuable minutes where you could be taking action *right now.*

More weight, less energy, ill health – is this really how you want things to be? With a small-steps approach you could be making real progress with your health and energy levels starting now.

As you continue reading I want you to repeat this mantra to yourself over and over again: *Doing on any level is better than thinking about going big. Doing on any level is better than thinking about going big. Doing is better than thinking. Doing is better than thinking…*

Phew, that feels better! Now let's get started.

## GET YOUR BODY OUT OF DEBT

Let's start with an exercise example. Think of your low-energy, unhealthy body as a credit card loaded with debt. As you look back at the past several months and years of careless spending you're amazed at how easy it was to blindly exceed your limit.

You're surprised and a little ashamed of how much you've managed to spend without really thinking about it. You didn't imagine it could add up so fast. Not only does the situation feel rotten, but now you have to figure out a way to manage the debt or things will only get worse.

Surprise, surprise, it will be a lot more difficult to pay down the debt than it was to rack it up. #@$%! *Sound familiar?*

Perhaps you depended on your credit because you didn't have a whole lot of extra money kicking around, so it stands to reason that repayment of the debt will require a little discipline. Given these circumstances, which debt reduction strategy would make best sense to you?

1. Occasionally drop a large lump sum of money onto your credit card when you have extra cash kicking around.

2. Wait to win the lottery, and while living in that fantasy do nothing to improve your situation. In fact, you make it worse.

3. Commit to regular smaller payments every week based on what your budget can handle.

## ALL IN GOOD TIME

If your low-energy, unhealthy body is the painfully maxed-out credit card you wish you'd never lost control of, think of your available time as the payments you need to make in order to get rid of the debt. How you manage those payments could mean the difference between reducing your debt or living with the challenge of high interest rates and poor credit ratings for the rest of your life.

Equally, how you manage your time could mean the difference between finally prioritizing health or continually chasing for change in a low-energy, unhealthy body.

Option number one – lump sum payments – could make a dent in your debt if you're lucky, but with so much time between payments and low cash flow to begin with you risk spending the savings before you get to the bank. Or worse yet, you may lose discipline for your debt reduction plan altogether.

Now apply the same logic to mending your low-energy, unhealthy body. You can wait until your schedule allows enough time and energy for a decent, lung-and-muscle-busting workout, but if that takes place only every week or so results will be lost between efforts and you'll be frustrated from lack of results.

Not only that, but you'll risk being sore and tired every time you work out and likely lose interest before long.

Scenario number two may sound like a joke, but you'd be surprised at how many people actually plan to win the lottery to solve their financial woes. The chances of that happening are about as likely as you getting the answer to years of physical abuse on the body through watching those crazy *one-pill-and-the-pounds-melt-away* infomercials.

Even still, there are those who continue with the fantasy, waiting for energy in a bottle, instant weight loss in a capsule, or perfect abs *in just 3 days*. It's like winning the lottery. Chances are slim, so I hope you have a backup plan.

## Look After the Pennies and the Pounds Look After Themselves

That leaves the third alternative: smaller payments every week based on what your budget will allow. Ten dollars here, twenty-five there, another fifty next week, or perhaps a steady two bucks a day. Dull and disciplined though it may seem (or perhaps because of it), this method actually stands a chance of bringing you success.

With small, regular payments it may take longer until you see results, but the consistency of your efforts has other benefits. First off, the small consistent payments will make a real impact over time. Secondly, you're creating a healthy habit around debt management.

Due to the regularity of your efforts your debt-reduction goal stays in the front of your mind and becomes a positive feedback mechanism that will remind you to adjust your spending behaviors to support success.

You'll start to look for ways to save more money. Eventually you may decide to make your coffee at home to avoid spending four dollars a day at the coffee shop. That's another twenty dollars a week to debt reduction. Good for you!

Again, apply that logic to your low-energy, unhealthy body. Just like your bank account benefits from small deposits, don't you think your physical health would benefit from consistent, small efforts at exercise, eating more healthfully or getting more rest? A short walk today, less sugar tomorrow, take the stairs on Thursday, earlier to bed tonight. Ten minutes here, fifteen there, more when you have it. But you make efforts every day.

All the small efforts add up to feelings of accomplishment, more energy, perhaps a smaller waistline, and before long you're looking for ways to do better for yourself, add in more time, or make an extra effort at change.

Of course bigger efforts would mean better results but only if you have the time and energy now!

Here's the truth: once you begin on your path, your time and energy will expand to bring about even greater success. Your small steps approach will create a positive feedback mechanism – a snowball effect – that will reinforce healthy behavior moving forward.

You could wait until you have enough time to do all those things "properly" or you could start today with one small effort at change. Start today. It's like *money in the bank* to coin a phrase. Brilliant!

Don't forget. Doing is better than *thinking*.

Small steps – the concept goes against the grain of everything you've read, overheard or been told about maximizing health and vitality, doesn't it? Well, if you've been waiting on the sofa for better health, more energy and a recharged life to hit you on the head you might want to listen to what I have to say.

Stop hoping for the ideal circumstances to arrive. Quit waiting for *enough* time. Give up the idea that motivation will materialize. It won't, and you can't wait any longer for some divine intervention to save you. You need a different attitude. You need a different approach.

> *A good plan implemented today is better than a perfect plan implemented tomorrow.*
> —GEORGE PATTON

## FOUR ARGUMENTS AGAINST *GOING BIG*

We've been conditioned to think big, dream bigger, make the big plans and get big outcomes, but going big doesn't always measure up. Big can get you off the couch for sure, perhaps even bring about short-term success, but it can also create frustration and overwhelm, and produce an atmosphere conducive to failure. Consider the following points of view.

### 1. Competence versus Challenge

When my nephew was not quite four years old I recall watching him struggle with trying to tie his shoelaces. His three-and-a-half-year-old brain wasn't yet able to coordinate the sequence required and his chubby fingers couldn't quite handle the flimsy laces.

He became agitated and frustrated, eventually breaking into tears at the realization that he wasn't going to achieve this goal today. Later that day as we prepared to head outdoors he slipped into another pair of sneakers and nimbly flipped the Velcro fasteners into place. Different skill set, 100 percent success.

When creating a goal of your own it's important to set yourself up for *shoe-tying success* by striking a healthy balance between your level of competence with a task and the degree of challenge associated with it.

If your goal is so big that achieving it will be met only through an excess of torment and tears, it may be too challenging to be enjoyable or achievable.

A few years ago I decided I wanted to learn how to ski. I've been an avid snowboarder since the 90s and assumed I'd pick up skiing quickly, so on my first ski outing I foolishly followed my very capable friends down runs that were far too steep and deep for me.

After numerous yard-sale wipeouts and a vastly bruised ego I reluctantly left my friends to their expert runs and snowplowed my way to the green runs. What was I thinking?

On those flat, groomed slopes I was able to shush my way down the runs, skis edging wonderfully, poles planting effortlessly just like a perky ski school expert. Without any real speed or challenge though, I soon became bored with the ease of it. I also felt quite unsatisfied regularly racing *and beating* the wee-ski kids to the bottom. Well, they *were* only five years old.

You see, too much challenge is one thing but total boredom is another. If your goal is so straightforward that it takes hardly any effort to execute, the lack of challenge could put you at risk of losing interest before you see results.

I found the right balance between challenge and competence on the intermediate blue runs. They were steep and challenging enough to make me work at my skills with neither terror nor boredom as my ski buddy.

The beauty of initiating your new goal with smaller steps is that you get to experience some success along with immediate and more accurate feedback as to whether you are really progressing on the right path toward your goal or not.

## 2. Decision Paralysis

Change brings about uncertainty, so when you're embarking on a new challenge such as starting an exercise program or changing your eating habits there is much to be said about keeping it simple.

In their book *Switch: How to Change Things When Change Is Hard*, Chip and Dan Heath talk about decision paralysis as the difficulty or inability to make a decision when there are too many options to choose from.

They share a number of examples where this was proven to be true. One such scenario took place at a gourmet food store where store managers had set up a jam sampling display, one day with six jams to taste and the next with twenty-four jams. Not surprisingly, the twenty-four-jam display attracted more tasters, but when it came time to buy they were overwhelmed and couldn't make a decision. The six-jam tasters were ten times more likely to buy a jar of jam!

As you look ahead to the new you and all the changes that need to take place in order to help you reach your goal of more energy, better health, less weight, fill-in-the-blanks, you may feel a similar paralysis.

*I need to start exercising! Time to get a gym membership. If I get a gym membership which gym should I choose, the one close to work or the one in my neighborhood close to home? I've always wanted to try cycle classes. Maybe I should look for a place where I can do that? Or I could join a running group and plan to enter a race in a few months? How far, 5K, 10K…maybe a triathlon? I hear running is a great way to get lean quickly… but so is weight training. I could hire a personal trainer! Maybe I should hire a nutritionist first? Before I do that I should see if either is covered on my health plan. But first I should get a new pair of exercise shoes. There are so many to choose from these days, I wonder which is best? And clothes, I need clothes! Someone was telling me about this great new line of affordable workout wear. Who was that again?*

When faced with this kind of indecision we'll default to what we know best, and for so many people inactivity and professional level couch-potato status is what we know.

You're still on the sofa trying to decide what to do aren't you? Quit thinking so much. Just put on any old pair of shoes and ponder the possibilities as you walk around the neighborhood for fifteen minutes. In the words of mighty Nike, just do it!

## 3. Eating the Elephant

*How do you eat an elephant? One bite at a time.* You're likely familiar with the saying, but how often do you apply it to your own circumstances?

Overweight, out of shape, unhappy, tired all the time and too busy to do anything about it...*what do I do now?* It would feel great to finally conquer the beast, but if the goal ahead is so mammoth that you can't quite figure out where to start you likely won't. Overwhelm and procrastination are common reactions when you take on more than you can reasonably or comfortably manage.

Insecurity creeps in, the negative self-talk begins chattering away in your head and before long you're talking yourself out of action. *I can't do this! What was I thinking? I'm not committed enough, strong enough, capable enough....blah, blah, blah.*

Here we go again. In your frustration you decide to never begin, put it off until the last possible moment or engage with less than full effort.

This is when you have to think of the goal as the elephant on the dining table. If the elephant were tonight's dinner, there is no way you would be able to eat the whole thing in one sitting!

If your goal is to lose forty pounds, you'll overwhelm yourself right back on to the sofa if you start thinking of *all* the calories you'll need to burn (140,000 to be exact) and how much exercise it will take to burn even a fraction of that.

You still have to get there one pound at a time, so if you focus on what you need to do each week to simply achieve that pound, the elephant will get eaten before you know it. Create a plan that brings success one exercise session at a time, one meal at a time, one day at a time.

Small bites, small steps. Same diff.

## 4. Psychological Hedonism

Psychological hedonism is the theory that all human choice is motivated by a desire to seek out pleasure and avoid pain. When faced with a task we're not particularly looking forward to, it's common to experience a rush of negative emotions – fear, anxiety, frustration, guilt, shame, anger – associated with it.

The magnitude of those feelings can vary depending on the nature of the task but one thing is certain: when we're feeling those feelings we want to get away from them as quickly as possible.

You vow to start a diet tomorrow.
You agree to start running with some co-workers at lunch.
You decide to clean the office on the weekend.
You need to sit down and create a financial plan.
You want to apply for your MBA.

Whatever your challenge, if you're not excited about it, bad feelings will arise as you get closer to implementation. You may feel shame that you let your eating get out of control, or fear that you won't be able to keep up with the others on the run.

You could feel frustration that you have to blow a perfectly good Saturday to clean the office. You might feel guilty because you haven't been responsible with your finances, or anxious that you won't get accepted to school. And there may be a whole host of other past experiences or beliefs dragging any or all of these tasks to the ground.

When those bad feelings crop up the inner voice perks up, *Oooo I don't like this. What can I do right now to make myself feel better?*

Your voice of preservation comes back to you and says: *If you get away from this task, you'll feel better sooner.*

By avoiding the task you choose short-term mood repair in favor of longer-term goal pursuit. It's a common reaction but let me ask you: where is that going to get you?

Now I'll admit that it's as easy to dislike a small task as it is a big one. Down-sizing your full-fat, double-whip mocha to a non-fat latte can bring as much displeasure in the moment as cutting out fat from your diet altogether, but let's reframe.

Take that elephant and cut it up. Attack the big painful goal through smaller, *more pleasurable* efforts instead of painting your entire energy makeover with one dreary, dismal coat of elephant-grey.

Eat better, exercise more, get organized, make a plan but break it all down to smaller less objectionable pieces of the dreaded whole.

Think about it. The task can be adequately down-sized such that you're able to get away from the dreaded feelings by actually completing the task. After a while the rewards will make each small step worthwhile. Hooray for you!

There's pleasure in that. I know it!

## Dream BIG but Start Small

I'm not saying you shouldn't strive toward bigger objectives with your health and energy plan, I'm just suggesting you start at a level you can sustain and then build from there.

Your goal may well be to exercise four times per week for an hour each time, and get your nutrition to *mostly healthy*. Heck, maybe you want to quit smoking too? Those are all great goals to get after. Just start responsibly.

Action doesn't need to happen in giant leaps to qualify as success. You want more energy and you can get that by simply taking small steps *every day* in one or two key energy-boosting areas of your life. The energy will trickle in slowly at first but it will be more than you had.

Let's face it, you likely don't have a lot of free time right now anyway and if you do you probably don't have the energy or motivation to go big out of the gate, so the decision should be easy.

To gain energy now, I'd much rather you take a five-minute walk *every day* than a two-hour hike once a month.

You'll have more long-term nutrition success if you cut out one little daily food vice like your morning muffin or afternoon soda than if you deprive yourself of every food you enjoy.

And going to bed twenty minutes earlier every week night will make a bigger impact on your everyday energy than a catch-up sleep-in on Sunday morning. What good is one mammoth effort at change if you get to it only every now and again?

The first step is small steps. After that you just repeat the steps day after day, week after week, until they become a welcome part of your routine. Your energy will start to improve if the efforts you make are even slightly larger than what you normally do. Trust me on this. *Less is more.*

---

*Habits are first cobwebs, then cables.*
—SPANISH PROVERB

---

You want this, right? You want a healthier, energy-filled, feel-great-again life, so make a decision. Decide that you're worth the small, daily investment of time and energy. Adopt a *Whatever It Takes* attitude and take a step. The initial steps need to be small so you have a greater likelihood of getting to them before that little voice in your head starts spouting excuses. If you stick with small steps, *the cobweb* won't break and you won't be able to reasonably say you have no time or energy.

With small steps you'll be motivated to move. Before the first *I'll do it tomorrow* even percolates from your gray matter you'll already have done what you set out to do!

Create a daily habit around a workable plan. As your consistent efforts bring forth real results watch your attitude shift from *I can't do this*, to *LOOK AT ME GO!*

You SO rock!

## CHARGE!

There are so many ways that you can effectively add energy to your day. The obvious energy boosters come through physical means: what you eat and drink, how you care for your health, and how much rest you get. You can also heighten your energy through emotional and social means: how you interact with people, how you address your stress, what you do for fun, and what you do to recharge. Let's not wait to get started, all right?

I want you to get energy *now* and not once you've finished reading the entire book, so I'm going to share some simple ideas that you can implement immediately and that you'll be able to build on as you continue through the book.

If you're a list maker like me, you know the best thing about creating a to-do list is checking items off the list when they're done.

We make our list to remind us of all the important things we need to get done that day, so why not create a special list and add yourself to it?

Last year I published an accountability journal called *GOT TO IT* with a daily checklist system that achieves just that. I'll share the idea here.

Prioritize a few minutes each morning to connect with your self-care purpose for the day. Grab your own journal or a notebook, date the top of the page, and make your list with a check box beside your item: ☐.

For example…

Today I will make a small step at:

| | | |
|---|---|---|
| **Purposeful physical activity:** | walk for 10 minutes at lunch | ☐ |
| **Healthy eating effort:** | watch my portion sizes at meals | ☐ |
| **8 glasses of H$_2$0:** | ✓✓ (add a check for each 8 ounce glass) | ☐ |
| **Better relaxation:** | take my lunch break away from my desk | ☐ |
| **More rest:** | get to bed 30 minutes earlier tonight | ☐ |

These examples focus on your physical health as a starting point. Feel free to add to the list or modify the entries to suit your specific goals. Keep it simple, keep daily steps manageable, and make sure you check off your goal once you get to it!

## GOT TO IT ☑

By creating your list each morning, you'll gain in two ways: 1) your self-care goals will actually make it on to your to-do list and won't be something you attempt to fit in once everything else is done, and 2) they'll be front-of-mind first thing in the morning, so you can begin executing right away. This will give you a greater chance of completing them.

Chart your progress as you go, and celebrate your success one step at a time, because that's all it takes.

## WHATEVER IT TAKES
### (*Small Steps Quantified*)

> If you want some focused guidance then visit www.gottoit.ca to see how I do it. This GOT TO IT journal will help you to plan and implement small steps toward realizing your goals through the day and then allow you to acknowledge your own success at the end of each day.
>
> ☑ **GOT TO IT!**

Let's see this *small steps* idea in action!

The other day I was short on time and wanted to skip walking the dog, but Lilly needs a walk regardless of my hectic schedule, so I decided to go for a half-hour quickie.

It was a gorgeous morning and the walk made for a good start to my day, plus we kept a pretty steady pace so I broke a bit of a sweat and likely burned around 180 calories. Mind and body nurtured!

For breakfast I had a cup of coffee with cream (for the record, I will *never* give up cream in my coffee) and opted for one egg on toast instead of two. I skipped the butter on my toast as well and my 170 calories savings was bumped to 206.

When I was downtown later that day I chose to take the stairs to my sixth floor meeting. I managed a brief burn for my leg muscles and filed away another thirty calories I wouldn't have burned if I had taken the elevator.

Since my car was in a great parking spot I chose to walk five blocks to my next errand, five minutes there and back, and I burned an additional fifty calories.

At lunch I found myself between a fast food burger outlet and a sandwich shop and I chose the latter because it had less temptation and healthier choices than the burger, fries and iced tea I was craving. With *that* lunch I would have consumed a whopping 820 calories, which is almost double what *one* of my meals should be.

Instead I opted for a chicken salad sandwich with extra tomatoes, a big bottle of water and a mandarin orange I already had with me.

Not only did I save myself 445 calories I didn't need but I felt quite proud because I chose the better option *and* it tasted pretty darn good.

I repeated that behavior later that day when I stopped for a caffeine hit. Instead of the large mocha with whipped cream that often taunts me I chose a small low-fat latte. Even with non-fat milk the mocha has 330 calories where as the latte has only 126.

204 calories in the savings vault! Even if I had chosen the large I would still have saved over 160 calories. YES!

At dinner that evening instead of having that second glass of wine I stopped at one. *Sigh.* That was a hard one, but I saved another 150 calories and prevented a headache.

Every choice you make in a given day (in this case with food and activity) either gets added on or taken off. Even the small choices.

By skipping opportunities to be active you miss out on calorie burning that can serve you in your overall caloric balance through the day.

By choosing less healthy food options or eating more than you need you add on extra calories that will either have to be burned later or will more likely be stored as body fat.

| ORIGINAL PLAN | CALORIES | SMALL STEPS | CALORIES |
|---|---|---|---|
| Skip dog walk | 0 | Short and brisk dog walk | 180 |
| No stairs | 0 | 6 flights of stairs | 30 |
| Drive the car 5 blocks | 0 | Walk 5 blocks and back | 50 |
| 2 eggs with toast and butter | 412 | One egg on toast no butter | 206 |
| Burger, fries and iced tea | 840 | Chicken salad lunch | 375 |
| Large nonfat mocha with whip | 330 | Small nonfat latte | 126 |
| 2 glasses of wine | 300 | One glass of wine | 150 |
| Calories consumed | 1126 | Calories consumed | 857 |
| Extra calories burned | 0 | Extra calories burned | 260 |
| Net calories consumed | 1126 | Net calories consumed | 597 |

In the *original plan* 1126 calories represents close to two-thirds my daily caloric intake. Since this example doesn't show an entire day's eating, there's a good chance I would have been way over my daily needs once I tallied my dinner and other snacks. The extra calories get stored as fat, and when you do the math you can see that it can add up quickly.

In the *small steps* example good food choices combined with small efforts at extra movement created noticeable calorie savings.

What if you adopted a similar *in and out* plan? Tomorrow commit to small changes similar to the examples I've shared. Do it again the next day, and the next day. Without going on a diet or engaging in big-effort exercise you could still find yourself down one pound in less than a week.

This small-steps model works with anything you want to be spending time at. Chip away every day and hit pay dirt in no time. Do whatever it takes!

## ENERGY NOW!

### Small Steps with Food and Fitness

- Stand up when you make phone calls.
- Don't go longer than four hours without eating something.
- Park a few blocks away from your destination and walk.
- Limit your alcohol intake to two or less drinks most days of the week.
- Instead of coffee when you're tired, have a glass of water.
- At lunch, eat slowly and pay attention to when you're full.
- Don't eat on the run. Sit and savor so you can relax and avoid overeating.
- Herbal tea counts as hydration. Sip away!
- Walk to the corner store to pick up that newspaper.
- If you must have that muffin, just eat half.
- Pack healthy snacks wherever you go.
- Take the stairs.

- Pick up the pace as you climb those stairs.
- Do five desk pushups before you leave for lunch.
- Run to catch that crosswalk light before it changes.
- Ignore the junk food craving. Crunch on carrots or an apple.
- Breathe.
- Smile.
- Drink another glass of water.

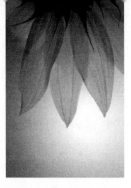

CHAPTER 3

# The Ten Energy Commandments

*If you wait for the perfect moment when all is safe
and assured, it may never arrive. Mountains will not
be climbed, races won, or lasting happiness achieved.*
—MAURICE CHEVALIER

YOUR goal is simple: small steps to great gains in key areas of
your life every day. Below is a summary of ten key sources
where you can get energy now – *The 10 Energy Command-
ments* if you will. I've created the list so you can familiarize yourself
with the contents of the book from the get-go and benefit from
better energy before you read the accompanying chapter on that
commandment.

Yes, each commandment has also been expanded into an entire
chapter with more detailed information, inspiration, and energizing
ideas to help you cement your new, energetic life. The 10 Energy
Commandments below represent vital mind, body and spirit activities
that will help you get energy now. Read each commandment, make
the effort to imprint the ideas as they apply to you, and take a step.

Thou shall not let yourself down!

## 1) Thou shall prioritize yourself daily.

*So much to do and so little time to do it.* You've already absorbed a fair bit of information that could lead to overwhelm, but don't fret. Remember, this book is all about small steps to great gains. This is the first commandment because the first step toward energy now is to prioritize yourself first…even in small steps.

If you don't make an effort to put yourself on your daily to-do list you know you'll be overlooked…wait, you already have been overlooked haven't you? Well, it's time then to make that extra effort and carve out just a little bit of time each day where you do something just for you. Make up your mind! *This part of your journey is already underway. Read Chapter 4 for more mind-strengthening information.*

## 2) Thou shall move your body every day.

Since you know that physical activity is so important for health, energy, weight management and longevity, *today* find a way to get to it, even if you lack desire or don't believe you have the time. Exercise energizes, and I guarantee that once you make it a regular part of your day, even in small increments, excuses like lack of time, energy or motivation will no longer be an issue.

If your busy schedule restricts you to less exercise than you're used to, don't wait for more time, start with less. Incorporate at least ten minutes of purposeful physical activity into every day.

**At work**
- Walk fifteen minutes to a meeting instead of driving.
- Take the stairs part way instead of the elevator.
- Get off the bus or subway a few stops earlier and walk.
- Park your car a good distance from your office.
- Drive part way to work and cycle the rest of the way.

**At home**
- Do crunches on all the commercial breaks while you watch your favorite show.

- Go for a walk after dinner.
- Do jumping jacks as you wait for the kettle to boil.
- If you already walk your dog, add hills.
- Do walking lunges down the hallway.
- Run up the stairs. Chase your kids if you have to.

Exercise less for success! *Read Chapter 5 to learn more about the power of physical activity for health, energy and self-esteem.*

### 3) Thou shall make healthy food choices *most* of the time.

If you want better energy, choose to make a few smart changes with your eating habits every day. Even if you hold on to some of your favorite foods, you can make big strides through bite-sized improvements. Here are a few ideas to get you started.

- If eating out is hard to avoid, pack healthy snacks for between meals.
- Down-size your full-whip super large mocha to a medium non-fat latte with chocolate sprinkles.
- Cut your portion sizes just a bit.
- Eat breakfast – even just a few days of the week.
- Be cautious of the little nibbles you sneak here and there.
- Choose healthy late night snacks.
- Skip the vending machine.
- Add in fruits and veggies.
- Trim the fat.

Food is fuel for functionality. Regular, healthful eating helps you think clearly through the day, keeps energy levels up and even assists with weight management and health issues.

Learn to enjoy your food, and know that healthful eating can still be delicious and satisfying. Fuel a new you one nibble at a time. *Read Chapter 6 for more detailed information and ideas to embrace healthful eating!*

## 4) Thou shall stay hydrated...seriously!

Why is water so darn important? Did you know your body is made up of approximately 50 percent of the stuff? Your body needs fluids to help with the digestion, absorption and transport of nutrients as well as elimination of waste products. Fluids also act as a coolant for maintaining body temperature and lubricating joints, eyes and air passages.

If you consider that 75 percent of North Americans are chronically dehydrated, then the simple act of drinking more water will make a big, big difference to your energy.

Drink water regularly to satisfy your thirst. Be sure to drink more water in hot weather or when you are very active.

Besides water, you can count other fluids such as juice, milk, and tea toward your daily fluid intake, but be aware of the extra calories as you do. Water you saying? *Drink up! Read Chapter 7 for bucketfuls of additional hydrating facts and fascination.*

## 5) Thou shall get enough rest.

Since when did sleep become a luxury? While you sleep, your body restores itself and repairs from the stress of the day. Inadequate rest impairs your ability to think, to handle stress, to maintain a healthy immune system and to moderate your emotions. Most of us aren't getting enough of it and we've become a nation of *working tired* holding on for dear life, hoping to make it to the weekend. Why not make your rest a priority for a few weeks and see how you feel?

- Get to bed thirty minutes earlier at least three times a week.
- Wind down your busy work at least two hours before bed.
- Before bed, avoid computer, television, video games, and work related phone calls that stimulate the mind and make it difficult to relax.
- Do your best to stick to the same sleep schedule.
- If you have trouble getting to sleep, try slow, deep breathing or relaxation techniques like stretching or meditation to calm your mind.

Get restorative rest and notice a positive shift in your mood and energy. *Zzzzzz's PLEASE! Read Chapter 8 to get the lowdown on slowing down. Start tonight!*

## 6) Thou shall stress less for success.

In the early 70s when stress expert Eli Bay opened the Relaxation Response Institute in Toronto, Canada he said that if you looked in the yellow pages under *stress* all you found were engineering companies. At the time the concept of physical and psychological stress was in its infancy.

Today, if you were to do a simple internet search with the word *stress* you'd get in excess of 540 million hits all related to stress management the way we understand it today.

Times have changed. We're connected 24/7, we work longer hours with less sleep and physical activity, we don't eat as well and it's taking its toll on our stress levels and overall health.

Stress is something that we're so used to that it doesn't occur to us that we could live without it, or at least live with less.

If stress is present even in small doses, it will negatively impact your energy and eventually affect your health. Of course stress is usually the result of a busy life and if you're busy you probably don't have time to deal with your stress. It's a vicious cycle that can be stopped with a small-steps approach. Breathe deeply, slow down slightly and *read Chapter 9 for a closer look at stress and your energy.*

## 7) Thou shall seek happiness.

Happiness has a direct link to a rich source of energy that no amount of exercise or healthy eating can match. It's true! Happiness is a big part of staying energized.

All you have to do is think about the last time you were sad, depressed, or lonely. You probably didn't feel like doing much, did you? For this reason it's important to nurture your happiness every day.

It seems like such a simple thing, but when life gets busy we sometimes just cruise along and accept what is handed us and then one day we wake up and think: *this is not what I signed on for.*

Do you like your work? Do you love the people you spend time with? Do you wake up and look forward to launching into the day? If any part of your life makes you unhappy, you'll expend unnecessary energy dealing with that pain – energy that could be used to advance your health, career and overall satisfaction.

Face up to things in your life that make you unhappy. It's not always easy and the fix may not be quick, but the results will be very worthwhile. Get content and get energy. *Read Chapter 10 for more on inching up the happiness factor!*

## 8) Thou shall be kind to others.

Imagine a world where everyone is just a *little* kinder. When you're trying to merge into traffic, someone lets you in. When shopping, you allow a person in a hurry to go ahead of you in the checkout line. You get back to your car and find someone has put money in the parking meter.

Rushing breakneck through our day, we so often forget that how we relate to ourselves and others is much more important than the things we do. Much of the time we hurry through activities so focused on the outcome that we miss the life-affirming interactions along the way. Begin your own kindness campaign by engaging in one small intentional act of kindness every day.

Why? Research shows kindness makes us happier and healthier. People who perform random acts of kindness report being happier, and when the acts are varied – holding the door open for a stranger, helping someone with directions, doing a roommate's dishes – those happy feelings last longer than if you were to perform one act of kindness repeatedly.

Beyond happy feelings, kindness is good for your health. Those who regularly help people have better mental health and lower rates of depression, and tend to have better immune systems. Kindness can also help regulate emotions, which has a positive impact on our health.

Go through your day with an openness to kindness. Walk with your head up and eyes open. Connect with people. Look for opportunities to engage and help. One small kind act a day is good for your health!

Attitude, gratitude and your health. *Chapter 11 is all about the energizing benefits of kindness.*

## 9) Thou shall embrace your passion.

I'm not talking about *that* kind of passion. I'm suggesting we all need to have at least one thing in our lives that we love to do just for ourselves. Unfortunately, when life gets busy we drop our passions almost as quickly as we do exercise, healthy eating and sleep – probably sooner.

Energy comes from doing things you love. Hours pass like minutes when you're engaged in tasks you're passionate about.

What fires you up? Artistic pursuits, sports, outdoor activities, time spent with family and friends, travel, photography, building things? What does it for you?

If you're not spending at least part of your week in the pursuit of your passions, you're missing out on a limitless energy source.

Begin by thinking back to the things you used to do that brought you joy. Next, think about the things you look forward to doing down the line when you have more time and energy. In *this* instant take a few small steps toward bringing past and future to the present. What a gift!

Start your own passion project. *Read Chapter 12 for an injection of spirit-lifting ideas and motivation.*

## 10) Thou shall exercise good judgement every day.

I've said this many times already. Change is challenging. And in the busy day-to-day rollercoaster ride that is life, the status quo – *or what we already know* – is vastly easier to wrap our heads around.

When fatigue and stress are high we default to what is familiar out of habit or laziness or lack of awareness. When fatigued we more likely default to the sofa instead of the gym. When we're stressed we most often default to comfort foods over healthier options. When work gets busy we regularly default to task management over business or career development.

We don't exercise our *best* judgement. We choose what is easy and tell ourselves, *Next time I'll do better.*

In the new plan, next time is now. Be aware of every in-an-instant decision you make that will bring you closer to more energy now. Start today. Keep at it! Do it for yourself!

*Ten Energy Commandments.* You can take them or leave them, but you've come this far so why stop now? Keep taking small steps toward the new you. As you read below you'll get a hit of *tough love* followed by an opportunity to create some positive energy for yourself. Remain open-minded. Good things are just around the corner.

## WHATEVER IT TAKES (*My Reality Check*)

*Oh my g#%! my life sucks!* It was early in the new millennium and I can remember thinking those words pretty much daily. I was working full time at a job that was no longer satisfying, I was building a part-time speaking business talking about life balance, stress management and health, and I'd let all three slide in my own life.

I was a personal trainer who had gained weight, I was stressed out, type A, hard to be around. I was unhappy. When my latest relationship with another mediocre mismatch came to a crashing halt I wrote myself a big old reality check.

*Why does this keep happening to me? I'm smart, I'm funny, I'm reasonably fit and attractive, I'm financially stable, I'm hard working…blah, blah, blah…*

I had been qualifying myself with this list for years, and while it was all true, deep down I didn't believe any of it – not really. I had to get to the core of why I didn't value myself at a high enough level to push through the fog and chase the silver lining.

I had to get to the root of my discontent and low self-esteem. In my mind I was a huge fraud.

I was an unmotivated motivational speaker. I was an unhealthy health expert. I was a life balance strategist who had no life balance. No wonder my life sucked! I started to see a counselor.

Maybe things aren't going the way you'd like them to in your own life? Maybe you've let your health slide or you're overweight, perhaps you're cash strapped or unfulfilled in your work, or you're wondering why you can't seem to stay in a relationship? Here's a bit of tough love you may not want to hear: if any part of your life sucks, *it's your fault*. There. I said it. Own it, and do something about it.

If you're tired all the time, it's because you don't take care of your body through proper sleep, hydration, and nutrition. If you have no luck with relationships it's because you haven't figured out the part *you* have been playing in all the failures. If you're overweight it's because you eat the wrong foods and you don't exercise enough. If you've got no money it's because you spend more than you make or you're lousy at saving. If you're not experiencing success in your career you could be focusing on the wrong thing. If you're unhappy, *if your life sucks,* it's nobody's fault but your own. *Ouch!*

If reading this stirs something in you or if you're feeling frustrated or angry, it may be a good thing! I'm not preaching this information from a self-righteous point of perfection. Not by a long shot.

If I'm saying it, it's because I've lived every one of the scenarios above and the only way out *for me* was to hold up a great big mirror and ask myself: **What is my part in this?**

Once I chose to own my part in it, my life began to change. Oh, I fought it at first. It was very hard for me to admit that through all the challenges and struggles I had faced, I was the common denominator in *every* aspect of my life that sucked.

Believe me, it's hard for me to be so direct — *and don't worry, I intend to remain compassionate and willing to help as ever* — but maybe the time has come to speak my truth a little louder at least some of the time?

Because on the flip side of that hard truth was the awareness I was *also* the common denominator in every aspect of my life that was great.

And when I chose to acknowledge *that* truth I realized there is far more good going on in my life than bad, so why not ride *that* wave?

The first step is to simply take responsibility for your life. 100 percent, no holds barred. Remember it. **The only person you can change is yourself,** and change requires your time, care, and patience.

Set the ball rolling. Face up to the changes you want to make. Keep your eye on the things you're already doing great and continue on with small steps. Do *whatever it takes*.

This loving kick in the butt was brought to you by someone who believes in the power of the human spirit. You *can* un-suck your life. I can help. **www.ifyourlifesucks.com**

---

# CHARGE!

## Write your personal growth mantra

Did you know that over 75 percent of self-talk is negative? Pay attention to how you talk to yourself. Do you berate yourself in ways you never would to a friend? Are you highly self-critical? If so, give yourself a little kindness, nurturing, and care. It's no *secret* that what we believe we achieve, and that starts with the internal messages we tell ourselves.

Make your internal messages positive and present-focused to bring forth real results.

Positive-focused means you identify the upside, not the problem. Instead of stating, *I will quit smoking,* frame it positively with, *I am smoke-free and breathe easily.*

Present-focused means you state your mantra as if it's already true – *I am wealthy, healthy, and loved.* Instead of *I will be...*

This power of positive thinking is an age-old practice that can seem hokey, especially when you may not be feeling particularly positive about certain aspects of your life, but when in doubt, fake it until you make it. Design your personal growth mantra to lead you toward the goals you want to achieve.

Affirmations are powerful. Thoughts, spoken words, and written statements are acts of creation. When writing your personal growth mantra it is important that your words be in alignment with your desires.

Develop a personal growth mantra that resonates with you and is repeatable when motivation and enthusiasm begin to falter. Here are some examples to get you started:

I say YES to success!
I give and receive love easily and effortlessly.

I am healthy in all areas of my life.

Every day, in every way, I am getting better and better.

Today I am healthy and prosperous.

I am filled with great ideas and the ability to bring them into action.

I love my work and it rewards me financially.

State it and create it! Write it below or on a separate page and post it where you can see it daily. Charge!

*My personal mantra:*

## ENERGY NOW!

### 10 Energy Commandments

- Create a daily self-care checklist and put yourself on it. Let it be the first list you get to in your day.
- Don't you dare think about skipping your ten minutes of movement today. Your health is as important as the work you put on hold.
- Go one day without sweets. Try fruit instead.
- Choose hydrating fluids over caffeine and alcohol one day this week.
- Change your sheets before bed so they're clean and crisp and rest-inducing.
- Take one thing off your work or home to-do list so you can gain a little breathing space.
- Tell someone close to you how much you appreciate them, even if they live far away.

- Look for ways to be helpful this week, even to someone you don't know.
- Embrace your brilliance. Write down ten things you do really well and revel in it.
- Recognize the value of small, consistent steps on your path to an energetic life.
- Go for a walk after dinner. Take your kids, your spouse or your neighbor.
- Add an extra serving of energizing leafy greens to your dinner.
- Exchange fifteen-minute massages with your honey. It helps with rest, relaxation and connectedness.
- High fives all around!

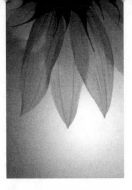

CHAPTER 4

# Taking Down the Time Bandits

*Time is an equal opportunity employer. We each have
exactly the same number of hours and minutes every day...
and no matter how much time you've wasted in the
past you still have an entire tomorrow.*
—DENIS WAITLEY

WHEN life gets busy it's easy to exclude everything but
putting out fires and dealing with to-do's. *Time for me?
I'll get to it when I'm not so crazy at work* or *I'll get to it
when I'm not so busy driving the kids around to their activities* or *I'll get
to it when I'm not so darn tired!*

In the process of taking care of everything and everyone else,
your own health and enjoyment of life gets neglected. And the time
doesn't seem to materialize, does it? So, how do we break the cycle?

## IT'S A MATTER OF PRIORITY

Most of the items we have on our to-do lists are often worth getting
to more for the outcome they will achieve than the process of doing

them. We don't always love *tackling* the tasks, we love striking them off the list.

For instance, it's good for my business and I love how it feels to be up to date on my bookkeeping and accounting but on most days I'd rather stick bamboo shoots under my fingernails than sort through receipts and reconcile expense claims.

Many of my past personal training clients would tell me they dreaded coming to their exercise sessions but always felt great when they were done.

And as my mother said to me so many times as I was growing up, *I don't care if you don't like your vegetables. They're good for you!*

If you wish to finally realize your health and energy goals then look at your self-care priorities with fresh eyes trained toward productivity and success rather than procrastination and mediocrity. Look for ways to make small changes.

*I'm all for it, Michelle, but I don't have the time!* I hear that a lot from busy people like you but I can only accept it to a point. Because really, when it comes down to it, it's not about time.

Well, it is to a degree, but be honest. You always seem to find time for things you really want to do, so in most situations your decisions come down to simple prioritization. Let's explore that.

## LOOK AT THE TIME!

Have you ever thought about where all your time goes? I mean really broken it down? We usually rush into the week mindlessly completing tasks and putting out fires without stopping to consider our choices. Yes, you have choices.

In order to find time in your busy schedule it will be necessary to examine where you're currently spending your time. I guarantee that with a bit of awareness and a few priority adjustments you'll uncover time you didn't think you had.

In his book *First Things First,* Stephen Covey helps us makes sense of how to prioritize tasks by differentiating between what is urgent and what is important in our lives. I've meshed some of his ideas with my own and suggest you also read his book.

## PRIORITIZING YOU

Call to mind your typical week. As you navigate each day you're met with responsibilities that demand your attention, tasks that need to be completed, and even a bit of free time to do as you wish. As each task comes your way you decide in that instant if it's important enough to get to right away, or if it can wait. You prioritize.

*Do I tackle this report right now or can it wait until after lunch? Should I send out these emails today or will tomorrow be all right? Can I afford to push my workout to this afternoon so I can join my office mates for lunch? I have to pick up my kids at school by 3:30 p.m. I want to sit on the sofa when I get home. I'd rather be surfing the internet than writing a proposal... decisions, decisions!*

### Have-to-do Tasks

Each day there are certain tasks you have to do so that your life will operate as smooth as possible. These obligations include work, childcare or anything that has a distinct level of responsibility attached to it. They include emergency circumstances and big deadlines. They include anything with a strict time line attached.

If you're bound by a firm commitment such as catching a flight, it takes precedence over going for a run. If you have to pick up your child from school it supersedes spending time reading or working. If you have a big deadline on a project at work, it comes before lunch out with co-workers.

**Write down the main have-to-do tasks in your typical day.**

Look at each of the items and ask yourself, *Would my life get chaotic if I skipped this item?*

If the answer is no, figure out how to reprioritize that item so that some of your emergency time is opened up. This will help you breathe a bit during your week.

The *yes* items are another story. If you don't take care of these obligations life will become very chaotic indeed. Duties like work and childcare are part of the responsibilities we have as contributing members of society, but if the have-to-do's are ruling your time, you may need to make some changes.

Are there items that can be removed from your list temporarily? Are there others you can delegate or tasks you can ask for help with?

Your goal is to meet the day's obligations with enough time and energy left over to focus on the *life* part of your work-life balance. So where does the rest of your time go?

## Distractions

Even during a busy day we can be guilty of allowing our focus to wander away from important obligations and into distractions like less imperative emails, phone calls, internet surfing, and other lower priority work or home related tasks.

You convince yourself it's all right since the tasks you're doing need to get done eventually. At work it's the non-urgent emails you respond to ASAP, the quick phone call that doesn't really need to take place today, the interesting research project that doesn't need attention until next week or the hallway conversation that goes on a bit too long.

At home it's anything seemingly important that distracts you away from the most important tasks of the moment.

You know you need to register the kids for soccer right away but instead you putter about with laundry, you make a grocery list, you tidy some more.

It's imperative you sort the tax information today and instead you clean the office, toilets, cupboards – anything but tax information.

It would be great to organize lunches tonight because tomorrow will be a crazy day, but instead you make some phone calls or surf the internet for last-minute flights to Mexico.

You jump toward these necessary but lower priority tasks in your day because they're often more enjoyable than what you have to do, you tell yourself they'll only take a moment, or you want to avoid other high-priority, often more challenging tasks.

And truthfully, all of your *distractions* can be justified as worthwhile ways to spend your time right now. But what happens to the tasks that truly need your attention?

Inevitably they get delayed to later in the day when energy is low and time has run out. Now you're stressed because you've run out of time, so you rush the process and don't give it your best attention. You may even end up putting off something fun so you can get it done. If this happens regularly, your life becomes an endless game of catch up.

Pay attention to how often you steer away from the important tasks of the moment. The quick and easy, low-priority tasks are like shiny objects that draw us toward them. *This will only take a minute.*

It's appealing to knock down a bunch of quickie tasks and gain that sense of accomplishment, but be cautious. Before you know it your entire morning will be spent ignoring high-priority tasks in favor of low-priority distractions.

You will gain a lot of schedule freedom if you pay close attention to the distractions you allow in to your day, and then simply choose differently. Be disciplined. Prioritize with purpose.

**What sorts of distractions pull you away from your important in-the-moment work? Write them down (and be honest). !**

As you survey the list ask yourself how you can minimize the impact of your distractions. For instance, I turned off my email notification so I won't be tempted to jump to my inbox every time something new comes in. I can always justify email as important, but it can wait until I'm done with whatever I'm working on. It's amazing how much more focused my computer time is as a result.

You may also consider how to make your high-priority *have-to-do* tasks more accessible and appealing right out of the gate so that *distractions* don't lure you away so easily.

As I write this chapter I'm sitting in one of my favorite coffee shops sipping on a non-fat latte. I'm disconnected from the internet so I'm not tempted to check in with email or social networking, plus I'm away from home and office distractions that don't need my focus right now.

The noise and people-watching are minor distractions in the grand scheme of things and I'm not at all compelled to clear the dishes off the table next to me as I might if I were at home.

The have-to-do's and distractions are what I call fire items because they usually have some level of importance. When any of them ignite you want or need to put out the fire.

It's important to recognize what sorts of tasks fall into these two categories and which priority level you're dealing with at any time.

If you prioritize with purpose you can minimize the number of fire items you have to douse each day.

A note of caution: when you gain that freedom in your schedule just be aware of how you redirect it. It can be tempting to pick up other fire-related tasks, but how about you invest a little of that time in yourself. And not by falling into the next category.

## Time Wasters

Let's face it, all of us need some time to tune out and stare into space, and often when we gain a bit of free time, fatigue usually makes that option appealing.

Unfortunately, the amount of time you spend on time wasters like television, internet surfing, video games, some magazines, phone calls, and emails will impact your efforts to experience success with your goals.

If you tell yourself you don't have time for exercise or other good things, check in with how much time you spend here.

If you watch more than two hours of television per day you've got time to exercise.

If you spend more than an hour surfing the internet for the best online deals, you've got time to cook a healthy dinner *and* make lunch for tomorrow.

If you play video games, engage in non-business related social networking, send more than twenty text messages per day or have apps on your phone with names like Fat Booth, Sim Stapler, or Beer Opener you've got time to read something worthwhile, take a restorative nap, walk around the block or call and connect with a good friend. Seriously!

Be honest with yourself here. I'm not suggesting you give up TV or other similar time wasters entirely, but if you keep telling yourself you don't have time, it's time to reprioritize. Growth opportunities are waiting.

## Get to Growth

I'll bet you have a list of tasks, goals and plans you intend to begin *as soon as* you've finished putting out the aforementioned fires, and... oh yes, when you have the time and energy.

I bet the list includes personal goals like exercising more or learning to play guitar. It may include professional aspirations like starting your own business or finally launching that new product.

Maybe you have plans to travel, quit smoking, get help with your finances or go back to school? Or perhaps you simply want to organize your office or improve your nutrition?

All tasks of this nature have a wonderful commonality of helping you enhance your life in one way or another.

If you truly hope to have a life of energy and abundance you have to commit time every day toward activities like these to reach and surpass your goals.

I call them *growth* activities because if you get to them regularly you'll experience unimaginable growth in your personal and professional life.

Professional growth practices include tasks like business development, taking a course, returning to school, creative work, organizing

your desk or filing systems, financial and business planning and implementation, or writing.

Personal growth practices include exercise, eating right, getting
enough rest, finding better life balance, enjoying leisure time with
family and friends, travelling or learning a new hobby.

Think about how your life would change if you could regularly
spend time on any of these activities.

## Get to the Good Things

Your health would improve in leaps and bounds if you could only
eat more healthfully, but you can't find the time to prepare healthy
foods.

Your energy would improve immeasurably if you could finally
fit in fitness, yet still you fail to make it a priority.

Your self-confidence would soar if you could finish your degree
or take that course.

Your personal life would perk up if you prioritized time with
friends and family.

Your business would grow if you took the time to organize the
books or create a sales plan.

Your life would finally be as you've always dreamed it could be.
If you could just find more time to get to growth.

It begs an important question. If you know that doing these things
will help you get ahead personally and professionally, why aren't you
doing everything in your power to get to growth activities at every
possible turn?

You can beat yourself up and call yourself lazy and unmotivated
but give yourself a break instead. There is a very simple reason why
we delay our plans, defer our goals and drag those resolutions from
year to year to year.

Remember this! All those wonderful things that await you in
growth require you to take action.

The have-to-do's and distractions are more likely to attack you
through the day, to draw you in by default. They will steal away time
so that the only way you'll get to growth will be if you schedule it in.

As you fight with all the have-to-do's and distractions you will tell yourself with best intentions, *I'll get to it when I'm done putting out fires! I'll get to it when I'm not so busy...tired...stressed...*

For this reason I sometimes re-title the *growth* category *I'll get to it when...* since we're always pulled away from it to deal with life.

Once the fires are out you likely drop onto the sofa into the *time wasters* category telling yourself you're too tired to get to exercise, or any of the other important and even enjoyable items in *growth*.

## Small Steps to Great Gains!

If anything is to change, you'll need to make a plan to schedule in your growth activities with as much certainty as any of your fire items. Here we go.

### Set Clear, Exciting Goals for Change

By now I hope you have a pretty clear idea what you'd like to improve in your de-energized life. And you likely understand the power of setting goals, so why not challenge yourself to make your goals happen?

Start by setting one or two goals for change. Frame them in a way that excites you so you'll be eager to work on them daily. Write them down and post them where you can view them daily. Better yet, share them with someone you trust.

Without proclaiming your goals you will slow your path to success by bouncing between multiple options. It's time to focus.

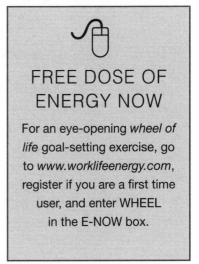

## FREE DOSE OF ENERGY NOW

For an eye-opening *wheel of life* goal-setting exercise, go to *www.worklifeenergy.com*, register if you are a first time user, and enter WHEEL in the E-NOW box.

### Anticipate and Plan Each Week

The next step is to put out some of those fires and find time for you. In his book *Power Over Stress,* Dr. Kenford Nedd suggests that much of our stress can be minimized through the simple process of anticipating potential challenges and working ahead of time to avoid them.

He says that one of the things that can make a situation unman-ageable is surprise. It's the unexpected that throws us off balance. Embrace this concept as it applies to your schedule.

Every Sunday night I open up my schedule and survey the week ahead. I do this so I can remind myself what's on my plate, but also so I can anticipate any challenges and perhaps even adjust my schedule to avoid a time or energy crunch down the line.

I may be reminded of a chiropractor or dental appointment I booked weeks ago. I may look at a particularly busy day and choose to shuffle things around to avoid the stress of too much to do and not enough time to do it. I could decide to block off some prep time for a project, or some time off for a lunch date.

By anticipating the week's activities ahead of time I avoid reacting to bottlenecks in the instance. My goal is to schedule only 60 percent of my working hours each day.

On a nine-to-five schedule that would mean that only about five hours can be blocked up with meetings, appointments and tasks that are non-negotiable. I include travel time in this as well. This way I have three unscheduled hours that will allow me flexibility to simply get work done, or to deal with emergency situations when they arise.

## Schedule in YOURSELF

Of course the absolute brilliance of anticipating for challenges and planning your week ahead of time is that you can be reminded to add *yourself* to your schedule for the week.

I'm telling you right now that if you don't take this critical step each week you will fall off the list (if you haven't already).

In order to get back on, you will have to put yourself there. Change can't happen in an environment of spontaneity; it requires structure that you create.

As you plan your week, schedule in your exercise efforts, your personal and prep time, your social visits — even your wind-down time at the end of the day.

I realize this may sound a bit uptight and rigid but I prefer to think of it as being disciplined and focused. The tasks you're scheduling are important and it's time you recognize how necessary your own health and wellbeing is to your energy, and ultimately your success.

Everything you undertake in a day requires time for implementation, and when you block your time in this manner you'll not only become aware of how easy it is to over-schedule, you'll be reminded to prioritize *you*.

## Get to It, No Matter What!

Now here's the clincher. When your *growth* tasks come up on the calendar, get them done. Go for that walk, make the call, get the work done no matter what your mind and body are telling you. Do that thing you have until this point always put off.

Too bad if your energy is low. Tough luck if motivation is sapped. And if your time is limited just do less, but do it for goodness sake… for your sake. Your time, energy and motivation won't improve until you push back against their ever present lack. It's time.

Sure schedules can be changed, but if you go that route try to avoid rescheduling yourself. You've had years of practice doing that and now it's time to take charge of your health, energy and happiness by prioritizing your needs for a change.

## CHARGE!

Who said you have to do it all? And for that matter, who said you have to say yes just because they asked nicely? When someone asks for some of your time, take a moment to consider your options. **Say NO** if 1) it's not among your responsibilities, 2) someone else could take it on with ease, or 3) you know you've already got too much on the go.

**It's time to find time for you.** Saying no graciously is one way. Here's another. Consider your current to-do's in a different light and ask yourself *What do I need to:*

Start doing…

Stop doing…

Continue doing…

Do more…

Do less…

Do differently…

## WHATEVER IT TAKES (*Learn to Say No*)

Stop thinking about your time as something you have no control over. Who sets the schedule? Who says *yes* too often when you know you should be saying *perhaps another time*? Who tries to fit just-one-more-task into an already jam-packed day until there's no time left for you? You do, that's who.

I have news for you. In some part of your life you are dispensable, expendable…unnecessary. That's not to say that you're not appreciated; you no doubt are. But that may not be a good enough reason to keep doing so much if the crazy schedule you keep is taking its toll on your health and vitality. You don't have to do it all just because you can.

*Reality check*. If helping someone else is hurting you, it's not helping. Read that sentence again. *If helping someone else is hurting you it's not helping.*

Your time – especially your free time – is yours to give. If you're giving so much that you're not able to take care of yourself through rest, exercise and other necessary self-care practices, maybe it's time to step back and say *no* for a change.

If you find that difficult, then try this on for size. When someone asks you for help with a volunteer project, a committee initiative, or anything that is not part of your job responsibilities, you do have the right to say no. If the person is persistent in their request, don't buckle to the *high-pressure yes.*

Instead put a great big smile on your face and repeat the following: *That sounds like a GREAT idea. I'll get back to you in twenty-four hours.*

Then walk away. This simple statement will buy you time to think clearly about whether this is something you can take on right now. One of two things will happen.

You'll walk away and decide that you actually do want to help and have the time in your schedule, and then you can say *yes* with a clear conscience, and there's nothing better than that.

Or you will walk away and recall all of the *other* things you've already committed to, the spouse who doesn't get to see you, the kids that are ready to disown you, and the gym membership that sits unused in your wallet. *It's okay to say no.*

Say no to their face, say no to their answering machine, send them an email; just make sure it says *no.* You're not a bad person for wanting time to yourself. Use it in the service of self to take care of yourself, have a little fun, and regenerate your energy. Do whatever it takes to learn to say *no. YES,* that's what I'm talking about!

---

## ENERGY NOW!

### Schedule in YOU

- Schedule six items per day (personal and professional) to accomplish. Everything beyond those six is a bonus!
- Practice being in the moment by listening better.
- Turn off your email notification so you're not distracted by every new message.
- Respond to email at set times during the day.
- Use the phone. It can be quicker than email and gives you a chance to connect.
- Make face time, not Facebook time.

- Schedule in some fun.
- During the day, answer your phone when it rings and save yourself the time it will take to check voicemail later.
- At home, don't answer your phone after 8 p.m.
- Allow five minutes every day to just BE.
- Make a two-do list. 1) make your to-do list, 2) block the time in your schedule to complete each item.
- Use your work coffee breaks for breathing space, not high-speed task management.
- Keep at least 40 percent of your working day flexible.
- For important tasks, time block your schedule ahead of time. Stick to it like glue.
- At the start of the week, schedule in your exercise sessions before life gets in the way.
- Set a timer to remind yourself to take a break.

# PART 2

## Take Care of Your Body

YOU'VE *MADE UP YOUR MIND* THAT IT'S TIME for change. Good for you, that's perhaps the hardest step you'll take in this journey.

Now it's time to get educated so you can live more energetically. The next five chapters will help you focus on your physical health and the abundance of energy you will gain by taking even small steps with your exercise, nutrition, hydration, sleep and stress.

I know it can be difficult to make your health a priority when the schedule is full and time and energy are nonexistent, but I challenge you to give it a go.

In pursuit of energy through physical health there will be days when fatigue will wage war with your intentions: *I'm too tired today, I'll do it tomorrow.* Please know that nothing will change if you don't, and fatigue won't miraculously leave you unless you push into it.

By now I hope you realize that my methods are different: do-able, hope inducing. Yes, you need energy to get energy, but with small steps you don't need much energy to get started. Fight the paradox.

I ask you to truly embrace the idea of small steps to an energetic life. Read the chapters, make consistent, small changes, trust the process and celebrate your progress.

You've primed the mind; now it's time to take care of your body. Heightened health, continuous contentment and endless energy wait ahead.

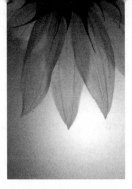

CHAPTER 5

# Fitness: Exercise Less for Success

*People say that losing weight is no walk in the park.*
*When I hear that I think, yeah, that's the problem.*
—CHRIS ADAMS

I KNOW you're tired of hearing it, but regular exercise truly is one of the best ways to live an energetic life. Yes, I know I write about multiple energy-producing methods in this book, but if I had to choose only one, exercise would be it.

Each exercise session you do packs a health-generating punch that feeds into so many aspects of your mind, body and spirit – so much so that if you're not currently exercising I have to ask: what in heck are you waiting for?

Regular exercise strengthens your heart and lungs, improves your strength and balance, aids in quality sleep, helps you manage your weight, decreases stress, prevents a whole host of chronic diseases, and makes you feel better about yourself, and it can even be fun. All of these benefits can and will give you the energy to succeed in all aspects of your busy life.

I know, I know, I can hear your collective protests from here. *But Michelle, I'm too busy, tired and unmotivated.* It's a tough one, isn't it? The very thing that will bring you an abundance of energy also requires energy, and you've got none.

Your goal to prioritize exercise gets further sidelined by a media-driven belief that the only path to success is to go big with your efforts. And not only are you sapped of energy, but you don't have the time either. It's enough to send you crying back to the sofa, isn't it?

Well, maybe you can get away with a little less exercise and still feel its energy-boosting benefits? How much is enough anyway?

The American College of Sports Medicine (ACSM) recommends as its guideline for basic health that adults engage in moderately intense cardiovascular activities thirty minutes per day at least five days per week *and* engage in strength-training twice a week.

Canada's Physical Activity Guide to Healthy Active Living recently modified its guidelines from sixty minutes of activity per day to guidelines very similar to ACSM. One hundred and fifty minutes per week of moderate-to-vigorous-intensity cardiovascular exercise *and* strength training twice per week.

The President's Council on Fitness, Sports and Nutrition advocates similar guidelines, which suggests adults should do *"2 hours and 30 minutes a week of moderate-intensity, or 1 hour and 15 minutes (75 minutes) a week of vigorous-intensity aerobic physical activity…in episodes of at least 10 minutes, preferably spread throughout the week."* Essentially 150 minutes per week.

Dr. Mehmet Oz – Oprah's now famous physician, and coauthor of the very successful *YOU: The Owner's Manual* and several other how-to books on health – believes thirty minutes of walking *every day*, rain or shine, is good for ongoing health.

Do you see a trend developing here? One hundred and fifty minutes per week give or take. If you can get moving for 150 minutes per week you will find health and energy in abundance before long. It seems simple enough, so what's the problem?

Twenty to thirty minutes per day – it's not much, but it's an awful lot. If you haven't been active, a move from zero to twenty or thirty minutes per day will take some getting used to physically, mentally and logistically.

If your busy life has transpired against your self-care efforts time and again why do you think this time will be different? It can be, but you need to understand what you're up against first.

**TRUTH #1:** *The fitness and health ideal you have in your head often doesn't match your plan, or the available time and energy in your week. Your life has changed and your plan for exercise hasn't.*

You tell yourself, *I'm pumped to lose twenty pounds in two months* but right now your schedule will only realistically allow you to exercise twice a week.

You say, *Well, I'll get up at 5:30 a.m. and work out before work.* But you know darn well you're not a morning person, so it's not likely to become a regular habit.

You lament that you used to be so fit without acknowledging that your career has grown and your available time for hanging out at the gym has decreased.

You swear you'll do whatever it takes to get back to pre-baby weight, but with two toddlers at home your time and energy have vanished. As your life changes, you need to adjust with the times. *Exercise less for success* – not forever, just for now.

One hundred fifty minutes of activity per week is a worthwhile goal to shoot for, and if you plan a stepwise approach to fitting in fitness it won't take you long to feel competent and confident doing just that.

But for starters I'd be happy if you moved for ten minutes every day instead of an hour every now and then. Think of it this way: ten minutes of doing is better than the hour you were thinking about doing. If

## How much exercise is enough?

There are documented guidelines for health and fitness that you can follow, but when you're first starting out, keep it simple. Your goal for physical activity is to *consistently do more than what is normal for you.* Choose activities that increase your heart rate and breathing. You should be breathless but still able to converse. A little sweat is a good thing. Need help? Ask an active friend or fitness professional for ideas!

thinking burned calories you wouldn't need exercise, but since it doesn't you have to get moving in order to get healthy!

**TRUTH #2:** *Success in fitness requires some effort from you. The first step to a higher level of personal fitness and health is creating the habit. Whether you're just starting out or working to a new level, set your goals and make a realistic plan for how you will get there based on the available time in your schedule today.*

This is a tough one since we're driven by results, and it's true they're slower to materialize if you're not exercising as much. Even so, you have to habituate to exercise before you can build on it. If your busy schedule allows for less exercise than you're used to, then start with less – just start.

If you start small, you'll be less overwhelmed by the changes, and as the exercise habit solidifies you will find more time, energy and motivation for the next level. I promise.

## Finally Fitting in Fitness

So, for the moment, forget all the guidelines and start with this mantra in mind. Your weekly exercise goal is to consistently do more than what is normal for you. I want you to really think about that.

**Consistently do more than what is normal for you.**

Exercise is about pushing your body just beyond its comfort zone. If you're currently inactive, it won't take much to achieve that, will it? In a strange way this is good news because as a starting point for exercise, then, *more* doesn't need to be much. So this is my physical activity wish for you.

If you're currently not active, from this day forward I want you incorporate at least ten minutes of purposeful physical activity into every day. Just ten minutes. On some days I'd like you to do more, but I still challenge you to get moving in some way every day so activity becomes a preferred habit in your new and energetic life.

A daily ten minute walk will make a real difference in your health and energy over time. In a few weeks some of your walks may extend to fifteen minutes, or maybe you will choose a walking route that includes hills or stairs.

Do you see how this works? Exercise less for success, yes – as a starting point. And if you consistently do more than what is normal for you, less will gradually become slightly more. More time, more intensity or more days of the week – all of which will result in more exercise success, a lot more energy, and less of you on the scale.

> **FORE!**
>
> Did you know that you can burn twice as many calories if you walk the golf course instead of driving a motorized cart! Not only will you be able to enjoy that post-round beer *guilt-free* but you'll improve your cardio-vascular fitness, gain lower body strength, and gain a new perspective on your golf game. Walk on my golf-loving friend. Walk on.

Start small, be consistent and build in increments. Add more time or intensity as your body tells you it's ready for more. It's small steps and consistency that will help you win this one.

## Four Steps to Exercise Success

You probably get excited about embarking on a new fitness plan. You think about the energy you will gain, the health improvements you'll experience, how much better those jeans will fit, how great you'll look when you lose the weight, how much more you'll enjoy looking in the mirror and all the attention you'll get from people around you. *Oh it will be SO worth it.*

With such big plans you're probably thinking ten minutes a day might not be enough. That's a fair assumption. More effort will not only bring about better results in less time, it will also ensure significant improvements with your health, so it's worthwhile to up the intensity on at least a few of your weekly exercise sessions.

That being said, too often we let our excitement for future results get in the way of our present-day planning and we leap into a new program without thinking it through and planning for success.

Without proper planning and preparation, you're sure to come up against roadblocks aimed at knocking you back onto the sofa. Let's take a few moments to think it through, shall we?

If your Level One goal is to habituate to ten minutes of purposeful physical activity every day, your Level Two goal will be to find three days in your week when you can build your exercise sessions to thirty minutes or more. These sessions should be more structured, with a focus on strength and endurance exercise that will build muscle and strengthen heart and lungs.

On the weekly exercise chart that follows, map out your Level Two plan. Consider the questions that follow and fill in your responses on the chart.

## My weekly exercise chart

|           | TIME OF DAY | LENGTH OF WORKOUT | WORKOUT PLAN |
|-----------|-------------|-------------------|--------------|
| Monday    |             |                   |              |
| Tuesday   |             |                   |              |
| Wednesday |             |                   |              |
| Thursday  |             |                   |              |
| Friday    |             |                   |              |
| Saturday  |             |                   |              |
| Sunday    |             |                   |              |

## STEP 1. Which days of the week are you able to work out?

Consider your weekly schedule and determine the best days and times for your longer exercise sessions to take place. Mark an X on your weekly chart on the days you've selected

Now I know you want energy and you want it now, but even if you have all the time in the world to exercise, I want to advise you to take a moderate approach to begin with. Keep at your ten-minute daily efforts then choose just three days – ideally with a day between each – when you will commit to a higher level for your health.

Next, consider the length of time that will work best for these sessions. Remember, we're shooting for a minimum of thirty minutes to optimize the health benefits of exercise.

Finally, choose the time of day your workouts will take place. Choose times that are least likely to be effected by meetings at work, your kids' schedule or your own energy cycle.

This can be a challenging step as you navigate your busy schedule, other responsibilities, and the knowledge that 5:30 a.m. workouts may not work for a non-morning person, but persevere. Prioritize and give up something less important if you have to.

Remember, exercise is no longer negotiable in your life. You're finding a way to fit it in, no matter what.

## STEP 2. Write down your physical activity plan.

To help knock down those pesky exercise barriers it's important to determine your exercise plan ahead of time. Maybe you'll run with a co-worker at lunch or attend a class at a nearby gym?

Perhaps you'll go for a walk when you get home or go to play squash with a friend after dinner. Whatever it is, try to choose something you enjoy that is also somewhat challenging, and write it on the chart.

With this step it is often useful to enlist a knowledgeable friend or a trainer to help you map out your best case workout plan, especially if you have no idea what you'd like to do. Keep things simple at first – walking or jogging, an instructor lead class, a sport you're familiar with. Determine precisely what you will do so there will be no questions or second guessing, just a clear plan with few escape routes.

## FREE DOSE OF ENERGY NOW

Walking is one of the simplest and best forms of activity and pedometers are a great tool to motivate yourself to move. A good pedometer tracks the number of steps you take in a day and can even calculate activity time. To learn more about my favorite pedometer and download your *Walking to Health* guide go to *www.worklifeenergy.com*, register if you are a first time user, and enter WALKON in the E-NOW box.

So now you've mapped out when and what you will do, and you start thinking, *I've been down this road before. I know exactly what will happen. I'll make the plan, and then when my exercise date comes up I'll come up with excuse after excuse. What if I don't feel like going?*

This question will pop up again and again, and it's the reason so many busy North Americans aren't prioritizing their health. You probably already know the answer but if not, here comes my *tough love version*.

### STEP 3. When your exercise date comes up, get off your butt...no matter what!

If you're tired, lack energy or are unmotivated, tough luck! Nothing will change unless you do. Go anyway. Excuses like not enough time, energy and motivation will always be there to sabotage your exercise efforts, so this time override your common response and do it differently! Begin to create the habit, even if you do less once you get to it. That's the clincher.

When your mind and body are talking you out of exercise yet again, tell yourself *I'll go anyway, but I'll just exercise for ten minutes.* Yes, you heard right. Do less. Just make sure you honor yourself and your exercise date.

Yes, the goals of these Level Two exercise sessions are to up the ante beyond ten minutes, but if the thought of a bigger workout is messing with your motivation, think small.

Give yourself permission to move for just ten minutes. By now I hope you've had some practice at those ten minute efforts so you know you can do it and it won't require boundless energy.

This way you have a chance to actually make it into your workout clothing and to the start of your workout where the likelihood of exercising for ten minutes *or more* is much higher.

To improve your chances of success at these Level Two efforts, you must first imprint the habit of structured exercise and then build on the length of time, intensity, volume or cross training that will bring real results.

And not only does exercise requires physical effort, but it also requires preparation and planning. You have to pack your fitness clothes, adjust your schedule, get to the gym (or wherever you're exercising), change your clothes, make sure you're properly fuelled and *then* do your workout. It's a bit more complicated than a ten-minute walk on your coffee break but well worth the investment of time and your new found energy.

If you become mindful of these first three steps, you will move closer to being regularly active at higher levels than you ever imagined. Once you make it to your workout, ten minutes often turns to fifteen or twenty, until eventually you've fulfilled your best case workout scenario or even added to it. But don't forget step four!

## STEP 4. Repeat all steps next week...for the rest of your wonderful life.

Yup, you need to do it all again next week, and the week after that, and the week after that. Exercise is not an all-or-nothing proposition. You have to do it to experience success and you have to keep at it to maintain your health. So set yourself up for success.

Fitness is indeed a life-long commitment but it needn't be overwhelming. Plan for three honest Level Two exercise efforts each week then knock them down one at a time. Before long you'll find yourself looking forward to fitness and finding ways to do it more. Won't that be great!

If your schedule allows it, do your first workout on Monday, when energy is usually higher. This way you can cross off your first Level Two exercise effort right out of the gate and you will have the good feelings of that exercise session as motivation to complete the other sessions. Awesome!

It won't be hard to schedule your remaining Level Two efforts in the six days ahead. Oh, and don't forget your ten minutes of movement on the other days. Now you're really grooving!

> Rather than put it off until tomorrow, make a decision to use today as an opportunity to add on an effort at physical activity. Do something active, no matter how small.

Finally, don't overwhelm yourself with the idea that you have to go big to make an impact. No matter if you're starting from scratch or have been moderately active and want to add on a bit more effort, your weekly physical activity goal is still the same: to consistently do more than what is normal for you.

Read the guidelines below for an effective start to your cardiovascular and strength workouts, then choose a few exercises to get started.

## HAPPY HEART

Your cardio routine is one of the key elements of your fitness program, so it's important that you get it right. Not only will regular cardiovascular exercise ensure a healthy heart and lungs, but it will provide you with more energy, and it's one of the best ways to manage your weight. Effective cardiovascular exercise includes any continuous activity that elevates your heart rate substantially from resting.

Great examples include running, cycling, step or hi/lo aerobics, elliptical, rowing or other cardio machines, swimming laps, continuous skipping or jumping jacks, vigorous dancing and fast walking.

WORK TOWARD
**2-3**
**times/week**

### How OFTEN?

Cardiovascular activity above what you normally do will provide a challenge for your body! If you've been inactive for some time, even short bouts of activity a few days a week will make a difference. For health gains make three times a week your first goal. If you've been at it for a while, you may plan to exercise more often.

## **15-40** minutes

## How LONG?

With continuous cardiovascular activity, time is a function of how hard you're working. Longer workouts (*forty minutes or more*) will necessitate lower intensity, but if you only have ten to fifteen minutes to do something cardiovascular, you can get real gains by working harder. The goal for each workout is to push beyond what you normally do.

## **70-80%** HR Max

## How HARD?

Intensity is a function of how long you're working (see above). Listen to your body. When you become sweaty and slightly short of breath it means you're starting to work.

If you're having trouble breathing or talking you may need to decrease your intensity slightly.

If you can sing a song during your cardio workout chances are you'll need to work harder. Singing requires a steady stream of oxygen and when you're working out I want your oxygen to be serving the muscles that propel you. Pick up the pace!

Push yourself just beyond what you're used to, and work toward maintaining that level for longer and longer periods of time.

I tell my cycle class participants I want them to work hard enough that they get a challenging workout, and not so hard that they don't want to come back.

### Been There, Done That!

Once you've successfully created the cardio habit, try different activities that continue to challenge your body and keep you interested. Weight training is a great option at any age!

## MIGHTY MUSCLES

Every year, from the age of thirty onward, we lose one-third of a pound of muscle. In ten years that's about five to seven pounds. Combined with an increase in fat weight as we age, a 2–5 percent decrease in resting metabolic rate, and a decrease in bone density and we're heading downhill fast. Ouch. Bad news!

Well, the good news is that resistance training combined with cardiovascular training is the most effective way to reduce fat while maintaining muscle mass.

Resistance training helps offset osteoporosis, guards against injuries and enhances other activities. Best of all, increased lean muscle mass will give you more energy day to day.

If the thought of *pumping iron* intimidates you, fear not. There are many ways you can add resistance training into your exercise plan with less effort than you might think.

MOVE TOWARD
**2-3**
**times/week**

### How Many EXERCISES?

If you've been inactive for some time, as few as five exercises will target the whole body. It's true. Since smaller muscle groups like shoulders, biceps and triceps will assist and stabilize larger movements by the back and chest, you can get a great full body workout by choosing your strength exercises carefully.

If you're new to resistance training, don't complicate things for yourself. By doing even one set of the following exercises to fatigue a couple of times per week you'll be on your way to better strength and body awareness.

### My Full-Body Five

1. Walking Lunges, Squats or Leg Press Machine all target the large muscles of the legs, primarily quadriceps (thighs) and gluteals (buttocks). *Feel the burn!*

2. Fitball Hamstring Curls or Machine-based Hamstring Curls target the muscles behind the upper leg and will also bring in

the gluteals for stabilization.

3. Seated Back Row or Dumbbell Row both use back muscles as prime movers but also engage biceps and shoulders to assist and stabilize. *That's a lot of fire power in one great exercise.*

4. Dumbbell Chest Press or Pushups target chest muscles as the prime movers and this time triceps and shoulders will assist and stabilize. With pushups your core muscles also activate to help you hold your position.

5. Abdominal crunches or any ab exercise that moves you through some range of motion will target your core muscles.

That's it. Five exercises that target nine key muscle groups: legs (gluts, quads and hams), back, chest, biceps, triceps, shoulders and abdominals.

The exercises I've chosen represent a small sampling of the options available to you. There are so many more to choose from. To ensure proper form and to make sure you're lifting the right amount of weight, don't hesitate to hire a personal trainer for one or two sessions to get you safely on your way.

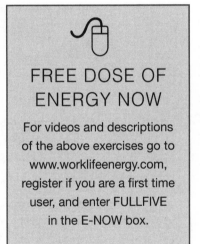

## FREE DOSE OF ENERGY NOW

For videos and descriptions of the above exercises go to www.worklifeenergy.com, register if you are a first time user, and enter FULLFIVE in the E-NOW box.

If you're more experienced with resistance training, adapt your program to include more exercises, heavier load or more days. Try to include two to three sets of eight to ten different exercises that can work the whole body.

## How Much WEIGHT?      to fatigue on each set

Weight depends on number of repetitions. Fewer repetitions means you need to lift heavier weight, higher repetitions call for lower weight. It's important to perform each exercise with a weight that challenges you to experience muscular fatigue by the end of the set.

If you're starting out, plan to do twelve to fifteen repetitions of a weight that will start to feel heavy around the eleventh or twelfth rep. Keep at this weight with the goal to always do as many reps as you can.

As you gain strength eventually it will be easy to get to twelve reps. When that happens, keep lifting until you reach fifteen reps. When fifteen becomes easy, pick up a heavier weight.

Don't be afraid to lift heavier weights. While you will burn calories by endlessly lifting a light weight, it won't do much for your muscle development. If the weight you've chosen feels easy after twelve or more repetitions, you're selling yourself short. Pick up a heavier weight.

Don't worry that your muscles will get too bulky. They won't. Over time you'll have nicely toned muscles and more usable strength in your body.

## How OFTEN

**2-3**
**times/week**

Activity above your normal output will provide a challenge for your body! If you've been inactive for some time, even one workout per week will make a difference. If you've been active for a while, challenge your body with more frequent workouts.

> If you are starting on a new program of physical activity and you've been inactive, injured, or ill, it's always best to check with your doctor to ensure a safe approach to your new plan.

## Stay Real

You can do this. I know you can, it's time, and you're worth it. Just remember, the only first step to realizing sustainable fitness and health goals is to make a commitment to fit it fitness – to create a habit around your plan, no matter what.

Chart your course and follow it even in small steps and this will eventually bring you results. Whether you're exercising, running a business, maintaining a household, raising children, or pursuing an education, time issues will prevail. And if you're one of those people who continues to wait for more of it to materialize, you'll lose the exercise battle before long and that's not part of the plan.

Remember, you don't need hours to change the outlook; you

just need to get started. Create your success habits ten minutes at a time. Yes! Exercise less for success.

## CHARGE!

I hope you enthusiastically read through this chapter so you could get all the exercise information you crave. I'm happy if you did. Now I want you to go back to page 88 and if you haven't already done so, complete your *Four Steps to Exercise Success* weekly exercise chart.

Better yet, when you access the FULLFIVE videos mentioned earlier you'll be able to download a copy of the weekly exercise chart at the same time. This way you can post your completed plan on your fridge at home or wherever you can view it regularly. Increase your chances of exercise success by knocking down a couple of barriers that get in the way. Your weekly exercise chart is one step in the right direction.

### WHATEVER IT TAKES (*Jackie's Story*)

Jackie, a past audience member, shared her struggle with finding time to exercise. She was a single mom to two school-aged kids and also worked full time as a paralegal at a busy downtown law firm. Her mornings were filled with getting the kids off to school, she often had meetings through lunch hours, and she usually had to leave the office right away at the end of the day to beat the traffic and pick up her kids. Apart from getting up at 5:00 a.m. (a move she simply wasn't prepared to make), she couldn't figure out how to fit in fitness.

After hearing my presentation on overcoming barriers to exercise something clicked for Jackie. At that presentation she remembered me saying, *Ten minutes of doing is better than the hour you were thinking about doing, so just get moving.* She started using her coffee breaks to go for a walk – twice a day, ten minutes each time.

At first she was surprised by how tired she felt walking *just* ten minutes, but then she hadn't been exercising at all and ten minutes was more than she was used to. She kept at it and within weeks she added stair climbing and even jogging into those ten-minute efforts.

Some of her co-workers even started to join her on her daily walks too.

She called her breaks *get moving* sessions to motivate herself to get to it on days she was talking herself out of it. A sign above her computer said **Get MOVING Jackie!** in bold print. On days she didn't feel like walking she'd tell herself out loud, "Get MOVING Jackie, it's *only* ten minutes!"

She began to really look forward to her exercise breaks not only for the energy the movement gave her, but for the sense of satisfaction she felt when she was done. She said the walks gave her way more energy than a coffee and muffin ever could.

Over the first two and a half months of her new exercise regime Jackie dropped twelve pounds, felt more energized at work, and even had the get-up-and-go to add in a couple of after dinner exercise efforts with her kids. She even started dating again. All because of her ten minute efforts!

No one says exercise has to happen in giant leaps in order to be effective. Jackie embraced the *Whatever It Takes* mentality and look where it took her!

## ENERGY NOW!

### Exercise Less

*Ten minutes? What difference will that make?* The next time you try to talk yourself out of small activity efforts consider the following. The average 170-pound individual engaged in just ten minutes of effort will burn:

- 56 calories walking 3 mph
- 129 calories running 6 mph
- 51 calories raking the lawn, stretching or chasing the kids
- 90 calories using the rowing machine, stair climber or stationary bike
- 146 calories using the elliptical machine
- 78 calories doing low-impact aerobics

- 66 calories doing Ashtanga yoga
- 90 calories doing hot yoga
- 54 calories enjoying moderate sex (FYI, you can add 10 more if you add 5 minutes of foreplay)
- 58 calories doing sit ups. I think sex might be more fun!

Let's say your goal is to burn 250 to 500 calories *extra* per day beyond your daily routine. Choose wisely and that can be accomplished quickly. If you need a more moderate pace a few ten or fifteen minute efforts throughout the day will get you there too.

Just remember, if you weigh more you'll burn more per minute of exercise – and less if you're lighter. To find more accurate results for your specific body weight do a quick internet search for *calorie burn calculator* and motivate yourself to do just a little more. It's all about small steps to ENERGY NOW.

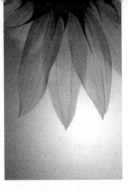

CHAPTER 6

# Nutrition: Fuelling a New You One Bite at a Time

---

*Tell me what you eat, I'll tell you who you are.*
—ANTHELME BRILLAT-SAVARIN

---

FOOD, glorious food! It's alluring, aggravating and oh so confusing. If it tastes good it's not good for you. If it's healthy it tastes like c#%p! Processed is bad, fresh is best. Healthy food is expensive. Fast food costs less. Good fats, bad fats, low-carb, no-carb. When to eat, what to eat, why we eat – it's easy to understand why healthy eating is a source of stress for so many.

Healthy eating combined with regular exercise is a big part of the Energy Now! equation and while both require a bit of effort to turn into habits, I believe the food change can be tougher for some of us to swallow. Why is that?

When faced with making nutrition changes that nasty D-I-E-T word pops in our heads and we default to all-or-nothing thinking and the belief that everything we love will be off limits.

Good-bye, potato chips. See you later, sweets. No more chocolate.

No more wine. Doomed to eat salad all the time. Flavorless food. Birdseed. ICK! No wonder so many avoid this healthy eating thing like the plague.

Yes, junk food and sweets in excess will wreak havoc with your health, energy and weight management over time, so you'll definitely benefit from living with less of them. So, what's the challenge?

Perhaps it's that you haven't found a way to balance your food intake between the less healthy options you crave and the healthful choices you need? It doesn't have to be all-or-nothing, you know.

Or maybe it's not so much letting go of the bad choices you love but being unaware of worthwhile alternatives that actually taste good. I promise they do exist!

It could just be that you need to gain a little nutrition knowledge to guide you on your path, and who can blame you? There is a lot of conflicting information out there and most of it is hard to swallow.

Healthy eating can be delicious, interesting and oh so enjoyable. At first it may feel like work but that's normal with anything new. Once you make good eats a part of your routine the energy and healthy feelings you gain will fuel your desire to keep at it.

Now before I get into the meat and potatoes of this chapter (no pun intended) I want to make it very clear that I am not a dietitian or nutrition specialist.

The information I share has been well researched and is based on the latest guidelines and standards necessary to make you a healthy eating machine. My intent is to provide you with enough sound information to make better decisions with your eating along with sensible small-bite solutions you can fit into your busy day. Oh, and I won't ask you to stop eating all your favorite foods either!

If your nutrition needs are complicated or linked in any way to health issues, invest in a few one-on-one visits with a reputable nutrition specialist in your area.

A registered dietitian or nutritionist will help you get the most out of your food choices and provide safe and healthy options specific to your needs.

In fact, regardless of your health status, you will always benefit from talking to a professional. Your nutrition needs are as unique as your fingerprint and a nutrition specialist will work with you to create a personalized plan that fits your lifestyle, energy expenditure and personal preferences.

## BITE-SIZED NUTRITION CHANGES YOU CAN SWALLOW

You'll be happy to know that I'll never suggest a total elimination of everything sweet, fattening, or carb-loaded. Not me! Food is life, and a big part of life is enjoyable eating. For me a definite non-negotiable is cheeseburgers. I love cheeseburgers.

Some people will say, *But Michelle, cheeseburgers aren't healthy.* But I disagree. Every food you love can be modified to a healthier, guilt-free version of the original and that is why a little food education can be so exciting.

As a starting point to better eating, you can energize your eating habits in small ways every day and experience success without the full deprivation of typical diets. While you're reading the rest of this chapter keep these simple ideas in mind. We'll build on them later on.

- Identify your biggest calorie-busters and consume a little less of them.
- Look at breakfast, lunch and dinner and reduce portion sizes just a bit.
- Choose lower fat options on foods like milk, yogurt and ice cream.
- Make fruit more fun (and balanced) with a bit of almond butter.
- Avoid fatty condiments on your sandwich or burger.
- Choose lean cuts of meat.
- Go light on your salad dressing, in quantity and fat content.
- When you're eating out take a good look at the portion sizes and plan to take part of it home.
- Eliminate sugary beverages.

And pay attention to your hunger cues. Are you hungry or eating out of habit? Make one or two small improvements each day. There are lots more ideas to come.

*Your body is your vehicle for life.*
*As long as you are here, live in it. Love, honor, respect*
*and cherish it, treat it well and it will serve you in kind.*
—SUZY PRUDDEN

## BACK TO BASICS

To live an energetic life you need to be fuelled by the right types of foods and a good balance of vitamins and minerals. Your *vehicle* will get you through life passably if you feed it low-grade fuels like junk food, sugar and processed meals but eventually you'll gum up your engine, your body will start showing signs of rust and decay, and you will slow down, probably sooner than you should. Maybe you already have?

The truth is, we want to keep eating all our favorite unhealthy foods and believe we'll be immune to the effects. But if you feed your body garbage eventually you'll be in the dumps.

*Instead, eat with the 80/20 rule in mind so you can keep some of your sinful favorites and be 80% great.*

—DAWN HART,
HOLISTIC NUTRITIONIST

What follows is a quick review of nutrition fundamentals. I think it's important to connect with ground level information as a starting point to reconfiguring your own plan. For more in-depth guidance take a look at the resources at the end of this chapter.

### Food Plates, Pyramids and Rainbows, Oh My!

How do you educate an entire continent on the basics of healthy eating when you can't consult with each individual face to face?

You create general guidelines like Canada's Food Guide and the new U.S. *My Plate* that provide basic nutritional information to the masses.

Both guides have gone through modifications over the years to educate as simply as possible on a complex topic.

Canada's Food Guide uses a food *rainbow* that shows all the different food groups and examples of foods and portion sizes in each. The guide is visually more complex than the U.S. *My Plate* but all the healthy eating information you need is there if you have the time to explore.

The U.S. *My Plate* has evolved from a very confusing food pyramid to a very straight-forward food plate that educates on portion sizes and how different foods and eating patterns can reduce the risks of obesity.

It makes simple recommendations like *make half your plate fruits and vegetables* and *drink more water in place of sugary drinks,* and that simplicity might be just the approach we need.

If you have the time and patience to navigate through

All three guides I mention here can be viewed online at the following web addresses:

**Canada's Food Guide:**
www.hc-sc.gc.ca/fn-an/food-guide-aliment/myguide-monguide/index-eng.php

**U.S. *My Plate*:** www.choosemyplate.gov

**The Healthy Eating Pyramid:**
www.thenutritionsource.org

Go take a look at them and decide for yourself – and guidelines or not, be sensible in your approach.

the websites, they are loaded with useful tools and information.

For another option, consider The Healthy Eating Pyramid. It is an at-a-glance pyramid that was developed by the Department of Nutrition at the Harvard School of Public Health.

The Healthy Eating Pyramid is in line with my philosophy that regular exercise and weight management are the foundation of good health, both of which are enhanced through healthy eating.

The food part of the pyramid builds on that foundation and shows that you should eat more foods from the bottom part of the pyramid (fruit, veggies and whole grains) and less from the top (red meat, processed foods and flour, sugary drinks, sweets and salt).

The Healthy Eating Pyramid doesn't try to educate users on specific servings or grams of food; instead it touts itself as a simple guide for how you should eat when you eat.

No matter where you get your nutrition information, be sensible. At meal times, choose foods that are *mostly* healthy, and pay attention to portions and hunger cues.

Fad diets and extreme eating may bring you results in the short term but they're often unhealthy and not at all enjoyable. Make it your goal to develop a relationship with food that is based on sound education and enjoyable eating that you can sustain over time.

# THE HEALTHY EATING PYRAMID

Department of Nutrition, Harvard School of Public Health

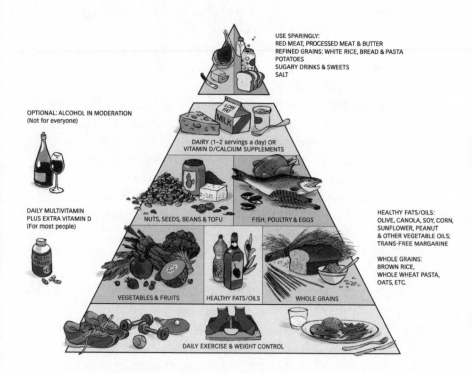

Copyright © 2008. For more information about The Healthy Eating Pyramid, please see The Nutrition Source, Department of Nutrition, Harvard School of Public Health, www.thenutritionsource.org, and *Eat, Drink, and Be Healthy*, by Walter C. Willett, M.D. and Patrick J. Skerrett (2005), Free Press/Simon & Schuster Inc.

## Nutrient Knowledge

It's one thing to know which foods to eat, and it's another to know why. To ensure maximum function and performance of your body it is important to have a balanced intake of a variety of healthy foods so that your body gains access to four key nutrients every day. The major nutrients the human body needs in large quantities are called macronutrients and include proteins, carbohydrates, fats, and water.

## The Three Functions of Macronutrients

| PROVIDE ENERGY | GROWTH AND DEVELOPMENT | REGULATE BODY FUNCTION |
| --- | --- | --- |
| Carbohydrates | Proteins | Proteins |
| Proteins | Fats | Fats |
| Fats | Water | Water |
| | *Vitamins* | *Vitamins* |
| | *Minerals* | *Minerals\** |

*\* Many vitamins and minerals are essential for a number of different body functions, as well as growth and development. They are called micronutrients because they are required in very small quantities in our bodies.*

## Carbohydrates

Carbohydrates provide the primary energy source for your body. They supply fuel for activity, are a necessary part of a balanced eating plan, and ensure proper organ function. In fact, your brain relies exclusively on carbohydrates to function. Good old dietary fiber, which is a carbohydrate, also helps keep you regular, and healthy bowel function is energizing in its own right.

As far as I'm concerned, carbohydrates are the misunderstood nutrient. Even fat gets a better rap. The low-carb, no-carb craze has people confused over what is acceptable for consumption of carbo-hydrates. They're an extremely important part of a healthy diet, and you should get to know them better.

There are two basic types of carbohydrates: simple and complex. Simple carbohydrates include various forms of sugar, such as glucose

and fructose, and cannot be broken down further. Table sugar, corn
syrups, honey, candy, sodas, all baked goods and pasta made with
white flour, and even fruit juice contain large amounts of simple
carbohydrates.

Unfortunately, diets high in simple carbohydrates can alter your
mood, create big fluctuations in your blood-sugar levels, lead to cravings and compulsive eating and cause weight gain in most people.
Too much of that good thing has been linked with a higher incidence
of diabetes, cardiovascular disease, breast cancer, and of course low
energy. Sugar doesn't sound so sweet anymore, does it?

The larger complex carbohydrates consist of chains of simple carbohydrates and include among them sucrose, lactose, maltose and starch.

Complex carbohydrates could be labeled the good carbs and they
occur in a wide variety of healthy foods. They are often high-fiber
foods, which improve your digestion. They also help stabilize your
blood sugar, keep your energy steady and help you feel satisfied
longer after your meal. That's worth chewing on!

## EXAMPLES OF HEALTHY COMPLEX CARBOHYDRATES

| | | |
|---|---|---|
| Asparagus | Buckwheat | Prunes |
| Artichokes | Oat bran bread | Pears |
| Cabbage | Oatmeal | Plums |
| Cauliflower | Oat bran cereal | Strawberries |
| Celery | Muesli | Oranges |
| Cucumbers | Wild rice | Yams |
| Broccoli | Brown rice | Carrots |
| Brussels Sprouts | Multi-grain bread | Potatoes |
| Eggplant | Whole meal spelt bread | Lentils |
| Okra | Whole wheat pasta | Black beans |
| Onions | Yogurt, low-fat | Chickpeas |
| Spinach | Skim milk | Kidney beans |
| Swiss Chard | Soy milk | Navy beans |
| Zucchini | Grapefruit | Pinto beans |
| Whole Barley | Apples | Soybeans |

When you survey the list of what qualifies as a carbohydrate, you see that it's not all about baked goods and pasta. The best sources of carbohydrates are whole foods that haven't been substantially altered from their original state – fruits and vegetables, whole grains, and even low-fat milk and yogurt.

These foods provide a healthy, carb-rich fuel source that will help you gain more energy, manage your weight more easily, and bump up your vitamin and mineral intake substantially. There isn't a dough-nut or cookie on the planet that can do that.

## Powerful Protein

Protein is a powerful nutrient, necessary for growth and development. Besides water it is the most plentiful molecule in the human body. It is found in all your cells and helps to maintain and replace the tissues in your body.

It makes up your muscles and organs, is used to manufacture red blood cells that carry oxygen to your body, and forms hormones and enzymes that help regulate metabolism and support your immune system. Protein truly packs a healthy, energetic punch.

Protein from food is digested into amino acids, which are then rebuilt into the protein in muscles and other tissues. Your body creates thirteen nonessential amino acids all on its own. The other nine we have to get from the food we eat and they are called essential amino acids. Protein from animal sources (like meat, fish, poultry, eggs, cheese and milk) are called complete proteins because they contain all nine of the essential amino acids.

Protein from vegetables, legumes, grains, nuts and seeds are called incomplete protein because they are lacking one or more essential amino acids. By eating different protein options in combination you can make your meals more interesting and ensure that your body's amino acid needs are met.

## EXAMPLES OF GOOD SOURCES OF PROTEIN INCLUDE:

| | | |
|---|---|---|
| Beef | Cheese | Peas |
| Poultry | Yogurt | Oats |
| Pork | Milk | Legumes |
| Lamb | Eggs | Tofu |
| Fish | Egg whites | Soy products |
| Shellfish | Egg substitutes | Nuts |
| Cottage cheese | Dry beans | Seeds |

As you look over this list remind, yourself that most of these foods have healthy and unhealthy options. Dairy products can be non-fat, low- or high-fat. Lower-fat milk or yogurt has all the powerful protein and a lot less calories from fat.

The same is true of meat cuts. Less marbling means a lot less calories from fat. If you want lean options include fish and poultry (without the skin) in your weekly meal planning, make meat cuts a bit smaller, and include more beans and legumes in the mix.

Lower fat protein consumption means more of your caloric intake is directed to healthy body functioning and not being stored as body fat! So, what's all this talk about fat?

## The Skinny on Fat

Fat plays an important role in overall health. Not only is it a major source of our energy, but it serves many other vital roles as well.

Fat helps your body absorb the fat-soluble vitamins A, D, E, and K. It surrounds and insulates nerve fibers to help transmit nerve impulses. Fat stores protect the internal organs of the body and provide backup energy if you haven't eaten for awhile. Fat under the skin is like insulation from the cold and the heat.

Despite its importance, most people have a love-hate relationship with dietary fat. You need fat as part of a healthy eating plan and it makes food taste so good, but it can also add a lot of calories to your diet and contribute to a number of health problems if you choose the wrong types. And believe me, fat can be very confusing!

There are two closely connected fat factors to consider. The amount of overall fat you consume in your diet and the type of fat you consume. You can't do one without the other.

## Types of Fat

We consume a great deal of fat in the diet through convenience options like high-fat snack foods and fast food. We also get it from fats like butter, margarine, mayo and oil that are added to foods, often in greater quantities than necessary. And when we eat non-lean meats and higher-fat dairy foods the fat calories add up fast.

In general, the healthiest fats for your heart are supplied by plant-based foods and seafood. Healthy fats?

Food contains a mixture of three types of fat: polyunsaturated, monounsaturated and saturated fats. Although one of these fats is not like the other.

The *good fats* (mono and poly), when eaten in moderation and instead of saturated or trans fats, can help lower cholesterol levels and reduce your risk of heart disease.

Polyunsaturated fats, found mostly in vegetable oils, help lower both blood cholesterol levels and triglyceride levels – especially when you substitute them for saturated fats. Omega 3 fatty acids found in fatty fish (salmon, trout, catfish, mackerel), as well as flaxseed and walnuts, are polyunsaturated fats.

The American Heart Association recommends eating two servings of fatty fish each week. Monounsaturated fats, thought to reduce the risk of heart disease, occur in avocados, nut oils and olive oil.

There are two types of fat that you should eat in moderation: saturated fats and trans fatty acids. Both can raise cholesterol levels, clog arteries, and increase the risk for heart disease.

You'll find saturated fats in animal products like meat, poultry skin, high-fat dairy, and eggs. They're also in vegetable fats that are liquid at room temperature, such as coconut and palm oils.

Trans fats are created when liquid oils are hardened into partially hydrogenated fats. They're used a lot in frying, baked goods, cookies, icings, crackers, packaged snack foods, microwave popcorn, and some margarines. So watch out!

Many experts believe trans fats are more dangerous to your health than saturated fats. And I say buyer beware! A product label may read *trans fat free* but can actually have up to 0.5 grams of trans fats per serving. These can add up quickly when the American Heart Association suggests we consume less than 2 grams per day.

## Sources of Fat in Your Foods

| SATURATED/TRANS | POLYUNSATURATED | MONOUNSATURATED |
|---|---|---|
| Butter | Corn oil | Canola oil |
| Lard | Fish oils (Omega's) | Almond oil |
| Meat, lunchmeat | Soybean oil | Walnut oil |
| Poultry, poultry skin | Safflower oil | Olive oil |
| Coconut products | Sesame oil | Peanut oil |
| Palm oil, palm kernel oil | Cottonseed oil | Avocado |
| Dairy foods (except skim) | Sunflower oil | Olives |
| Partially hydrogenated oils | Nuts and seeds | Peanut butter |

Your goal is to lower your total fat intake, reduce your saturated fat to less than 10 percent of your total, and engage in an overall healthy lifestyle. A bit of label reading and awareness is the first step.

## ENERGIZE YOUR EATING

If you're serious about having an energetic life you'll need to embrace healthy eating as a lifestyle and not as something you do once in a while to feel better about yourself or lose a few pounds. There are better ways to achieve that goal.

Below I outline four key aspects of healthy eating: timing, variety, balance and moderation. If you make improvements with just one of these areas you'll feel better, but if you include ideas from all four, watch out! You'll have so much energy you'll be climbing the healthy eating pyramid instead of reading it!

## Timing

Think of your body as a wood-burning stove. The food you eat throughout the day to fuel your body is like wood for the fire. And just like wood, it eventually burns down to ash, emitting energy as it does. Your goal with eating then is to never let the fire go cold, to make sure it always has fuel coming in.

In order to eat for energy you need to eat often: five to six times per day to be more precise, or every two to four hours. Three main meals each day with healthy snacks in between will allow for a steady supply of energy to fuel you throughout the day.

In the morning the *stove* is cold because all the fuel you fed it last night has burned to ashes. The breakfast you eat serves as the first *load of wood* to rekindle the fire. It's why breakfast is such an important meal. Without it the ashes remain cold, your body's metabolism is dialed down to low, and you will have less energy to start your day.

Once you eat breakfast your body's fire gets lit and you gain good energy to carry you through the morning. Good for you! Don't ignore the tummy grumbles you feel a few hours later though. It's your body telling you that the wood is burning to ash. It's time to stoke the fire with a healthy snack.

> Did you know that people who skip breakfast take in less calcium, iron, fiber and energy: nutrients that don't get replaced in other meals? They are also more likely to be overweight than breakfast eaters. Eggs anyone?

By the way, coffee and a big ol' muffin do not qualify as healthy. How about you try some fruit for a change? Add a little protein so you gain more nutrients and feel full longer. Try to avoid excessive sweets. Those packaged 100-calorie snack-packs, for instance, are loaded with simple sugars, sodium and very few nutrients. You can do better for yourself.

## Energizing Snack Ideas

- An apple, pear or banana spread with almond butter
- Carrot and celery sticks dipped in hummus
- Half a cup of low-fat yogurt sprinkled with granola

- Cheese on whole-grain crackers
- A rice cake with almond butter and sliced strawberries
- A low-fat latte or flavored steamer
- A handful of almonds and a few pieces of dried fruit
- A boiled egg on whole wheat toast (no butter)
- Half a cup of low-fat cottage cheese with fruit or apple sauce

**Snack-tastic!**

How about this? For one week replace your morning muffin or afternoon vending machine raid with an energizing snack and see how much better you feel. Small bites – healthy ones at that.

What these snacks have in common is that they all combine healthy carbs with a bit of protein, and where possible, lower fat. Snacks like these will give your body more usable calories and more energy than any amount of java and sweets.

Remember, your goal is to keep the fire burning. If the wood burns down to nothing over several hours without fuel, you run the risk of satisfying your big hunger with something convenient and unhealthy. Not only do you consume more calories in this situation, but you experience a spike in blood sugar levels followed by a fatiguing drop once the quick calories burn out. That's not energizing.

Listen to your body and learn to tell the difference between eating out of habit and eating for hunger. Use your watch as a guide and don't allow more than four hours to pass without nibbling on something healthy.

## Variety

By eating a variety of different foods in each of the main nutrient groups every day, you have the best chance of getting all the essential vitamins and minerals your body needs to stay healthy.

It also makes eating far more exciting. Use this as a chance to explore new foods and try new recipes. There are so many wonderful ways to combine foods. Learn from other cultures. Take a cooking class. Buy a fun cook book. I've listed a few of my favorites at the end of this chapter.

Variety truly is the spice of life… and your meal times.

## Balance

The concept of a balanced meal has become lost in our fast-paced busy lives. We're conditioned to grab and go with fast food or prepackaged, processed food that fits in our pocket for later. The problem with these convenience foods is that they rarely include all the important food groups your body needs. In fact they usually contain too much fat and simple carbohydrates and very little fresh fruits or vegetables.

In order to eat for energy it's important to balance your three main meals to include foods from three important categories.

### Color your world

My mom has had a vegetable garden for as long as I can remember. When we were growing up she always made a point of including several colorful vegetables in each meal – yellow squash, green salad, orange carrots, purple beets, juicy red tomatoes. I may have complained about eating my veggies, but I have to admit, our meals were pretty.

Think of your plate as an artist's palate. Include as many colors as possible to make your health picture bright!

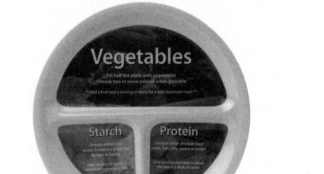

Vegetables and fruit, 50 percent

Whole grains, 25 percent

Meat and alternatives, 25 percent

The portion control plate shown above is the right size to help you visualize healthy portions. It is available at *www.stepscount.com*.

Here's an easy way to break it down. Fill half your plate with healthy vegetables and a bit of fruit. This can come from multiple sources like a salad, steamed or roasted vegetables, or a piece of fruit. Don't hold back on veggie portion sizes. They're high in vitamins and minerals and low in calories.

One quarter of your plate is for your protein source. A piece of chicken or fish, a small steak, sliced egg, tofu or other soy products are all great options. Try to minimize protein portion size to three to four ounces per meal — about the size of one deck of playing cards.

The last quarter is for your grain or starch. Brown rice, sweet potatoes, grainy bread, mashed potatoes or whole wheat pasta will help fill you up and give you sustainable energy from the complex carbohydrates category. Think of portions the size of your fist and no larger.

Add a glass of milk with your meal or a half cup of flavored yogurt for dessert to get some calcium.

*Life expectancy would grow by leaps and bounds*
*if green vegetables smelled as good as bacon.*
—Doug Larson

Don't be afraid to combine categories to keep your meal time exciting. Forget plain old eggs and toast. Scrambled eggs are delicious with spinach and mushrooms cooked in.

Your salad at lunch is more exciting when you include a few different vegetables. Try grated carrot or beets. Toss in some bean sprouts, chick peas, sun dried tomatoes, or artichokes. You can include salmon, roast chicken or tuna along with a sprinkle of toasted nuts. I sometimes toss in a bit of cooked quinoa or couscous and skip the bread.

At dinner try brown rice mixed with sautéed onions and peppers, or mashed potatoes and sweet potatoes combined. One of my winter favorites is root vegetables — carrots, beets, parsnips, yams and potatoes — tossed in a wee bit of olive oil and herbs and roasted in the oven.

At lunch you can still have that ham sandwich. You can balance it out if you choose whole grain bread and add tomatoes, spinach, sliced red peppers or some of your other veggie favorites.

Just make sure each of your main meals includes a protein source, some whole grains, and one or two servings of vegetables or fruit.

And of course it's always a good idea to fill some of your protein and carb options with dairy products or calcium-rich foods to help keep bones and teeth strong, especially as you age. Most adults need about 1000–1200 mg of calcium per day. An eight-ounce glass of milk contains 300 mg.

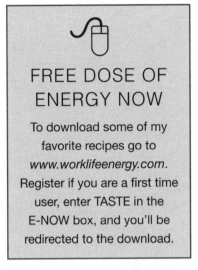

## FREE DOSE OF ENERGY NOW

To download some of my favorite recipes go to *www.worklifeenergy.com*. Register if you are a first time user, enter TASTE in the E-NOW box, and you'll be redirected to the download.

Good, non-dairy sources of calcium include leafy green vegetables, like swiss chard, collard greens and bok choy. Fortified soy milk is also high in calcium. So are baked beans, almonds and fish canned with the bones.

If you take supplements, choose one that contains both calcium and vitamin D since the latter helps absorption of the former.

## SIZE MATTERS!

Did you know that over the past few decades portion sizes have increased on most foods we eat? Not only have restaurant meals grown in size but bags of snack foods and soft drinks in vending machines and convenience stores have gotten larger and larger.

### Love Those Veggies!

You'll notice that many of my examples provide suggestions that add vegetables into the mix. Most of us don't eat enough veggies and if you want more energy, Popeye was right. Eat your spinach! Vegetables are a great way to add volume to your meal without an excess of extra calories. They're also packed with vitamins and minerals, are high in dietary fiber and add amazing flavor without adding fat.

Even the prepackaged foods we buy to eat at home have increased in size. Not surprisingly, our waistlines have expanded along with this increase in portion sizes, so it's time for a little *eating awareness.*

Eating for energy requires a close look at not only what you're eating, but how much of it you consume at any given time. There is a very big difference between serving size and portion size.

A portion size is the amount of a single food item served in a single eating occasion. A serving size is a standardized unit for measuring foods, like half a cup or six ounces, and is related to nutritional needs of your body.

That slice of pizza you buy for lunch is one portion size but likely closer to two servings. That 500ml (16 ounce) chocolate milk you just bought is two serving sizes. Most restaurant meals are large enough to feed two people.

Unfortunately, most of us will eat more when we're faced with larger portions. Mindless eating takes over. We eat too fast, we eat on the run, and we don't pay attention to our hunger cues, and this behavior is robbing us of energy and food enjoyment.

> *Moderation. Small helpings.*
> *Sample a little bit of everything.*
> *These are the secrets of happiness and good health.*
> —JULIA CHILD

Here are a number of ways to embrace moderation with your eating:

- Make sure your plate is not larger than ten inches in diameter, and never load the plate to heaping.
- Slow down and enjoy your meals. If you speed through a meal you're likely to overeat.
- Sit at the kitchen table away from television or work. When distracted we mindlessly consume.
- Fill your plate based on the balanced plan above. Put away leftovers before you sit to eat so you won't be tempted to nibble on extras.
- Before you go for seconds have a glass of water and wait. It takes your body about twenty minutes to register that it's full. If you rush into seconds too soon you're likely to overeat.

- In a restaurant take a close look at the size of your meal. If it's big, have half of it boxed up before you begin, or share the meal with a friend.

- Order a size smaller than your usual. When you finish consuming, pay attention to your hunger. Chances are you've had enough.

- Read labels and get educated on reasonable serving sizes. Just because you bought the package doesn't mean you need to eat the whole darn thing.

## Balance the Guilty Pleasures

It would be foolish and no fun to stop eating all the foods you love, so how about we strike a deal?

It's one thing to seek moderation with the amount of food you eat; it's entirely another to seek it regarding *what* you eat. Too much of a good thing is not a good thing.

If you go on eating all of the unhealthy foods you love in unlimited quantities your health, weight management and energy will take a beating, not to mention your self-esteem. I say we inject a little self-discipline into the mix.

The best way to keep eating the foods you love is to compromise in two important ways:

1. Eat a little less of your favorite foods.

2. Let go of less appealing favorites in favor of healthier options to free up calories in your daily meal plan.

## Eat a Little *Less* of Your Favorite Foods

Often our food choices are based on habit and a wee bit of self-indulgence. Maybe it didn't occur to you to order a smaller size? You love it so much you want as much of it as you can get, but how about learning to live with less?

This applies to anything you consume through the day – even healthier options. If you don't need a large, don't order it.

I used to always buy a large fruit smoothie from my favorite juice bar, and while it was packed with fruit and frozen yogurt goodness, I always struggled to finish the whole thing. It didn't occur to me to a) stop sipping when I was full, or b) order a smaller size. Then one day it dawned on me to order the snack size. All the goodness, half the size, and now I save money *and* calories on every smoothie indulgence.

- Decrease daily indulgences to every other day.
- Pack your lunch with a wee bit less of your favorite baked goods.
- Order a smaller portion or a smaller size.
- Fill your plate with a little less.

Tell yourself it's not about deprivation, it's about discipline. A little discipline with your food vices can go a long way to helping you regain health and energy.

Simply allow yourself a reasonable dose of what one of my clients calls daily *fun foods* and you won't be seeking out every sugar- and fat-laden treat on the planet. I guarantee that when you do get to eat your favorite foods you'll be rewarded with guilt-free enjoyment, knowing you've exercised some healthy restraint along the way.

## Let Go of Less Appealing Favorites

I've already confessed to a love of cheeseburgers, and I doubt red wine will ever be off my consumption list, but I should mention the compromises I make so my favorites can happily fit into my life.

For starters, when I order a cheeseburger I ask for it without bacon or mayonnaise. By living without those two fatty toppings I can happily enjoy the cheese. And I rarely have french fries as a side. I replace that calorie-laden indulgence with a big salad with the dressing on the side. Those two sacrifices easily save me 1000 calories or more and make my cheeseburger experience a guilt-free, healthy, balanced meal.

During the day I eliminate juice, soda or other liquid calories in favor of good old $H_2O$. I tend to do this regardless of whether I plan to have a glass or two of wine, but in the event I do, it fits easily into my day without adding too much excess.

When you eat out choose restaurants that serve healthy options so your decision making will be easy. Remember, healthy doesn't have to taste bad. Small sacrifices in some areas will mean full gratification in others.

What foods can you live without? Be ruthless in your screening so you can still enjoy your favorites.

## Watching the Waistline

Close to 70 percent of the North American population struggles with being overweight or obese. It's no wonder then that so many people have a strained relationship with food, viewing it as the enemy in their battle to lose weight.

While it's true that weight management is a result of calories in versus calories out, I want to caution you about obsessive calorie counting as a method for weight loss.

Yes, it's helpful to have a general idea about how many calories certain foods have, and to understand your own daily requirements, so you avoid overindulgence, but there are healthy ways to accomplish that goal.

It's far more important to learn the difference between healthy and unhealthy options, to create an enjoyable balance between them, and above all, to tune in to your body's needs and desires for food.

## Intuitive Eating

Intuitive eating suggests that tuning in to your body's natural hunger signals is a more effective way to attain a healthy weight than calorie counting or monitoring energy and fats in foods.

Before you start eating let your body tell you whether it's hungry. If you've had a proper meal recently then maybe you're reaching for food out of boredom or to make yourself feel better.

When you reach for unhealthy options ask yourself if there is a better alternative. If you simply must indulge in that moment, cut back on the amount you eat.

When you eat, slow down and savor the meal and take note of when you become full. When you feel full, stop eating. Get up and walk away from the table. Pack up the rest of your meal for another time. Tell yourself that if hunger returns a little later, it's okay to have a snack.

Pay attention to how your body feels when you feed it the wrong kinds of foods or eat too much food in one sitting. At the same time, notice how much better you feel when most of your food choices are healthy.

Weight management is about feeding your body nourishing food in moderation. It's about cutting back on unhealthy foods and adding in more physical activity, plain and simple.

The one instance where I feel calorie counting can be helpful is through small steps and small bites. If you consider that every pound of fat has 3500 calories, then start counting all the small ways you can eliminate unhealthy calories from your meal plan.

Or better yet, why not look for ways to burn an extra 250 calories per day through activity and at the same time find ways to eliminate 250 calories from your daily meal plan? That's 500 calories per day that will amount to 3500 calories, or a healthy one pound of weight loss per week. Look for calorie saving ideas at the end of this chapter.

Healthy eating is definitely one of the best options for living an energetic life, and it can be a tasty and enjoyable experience. Start with small bites, ask for help if you need it, and fuel a new you.

Treat your body well and it will respond in kind.

## CHARGE!

Increase your chances of healthy eating success by learning as much as you can about nutrition in general, and your relationship with food in specific. A registered dietitian or nutritionist will educate you and motivate you to new levels of health, energy and vitality with your eating. It's a worthwhile investment, to be sure.

At the end of this book I've listed a number of worthwhile nutrition resources that provide great information on different aspects of healthy eating. Arm yourself with knowledge and feel the power of eating for energy now.

## WHATEVER IT TAKES (*Valerie's Story*)

In 2003 my friend and coaching colleague Valerie lost a big part of herself and hopes she never finds it – 170 pounds of herself to be exact. She's waged a thirty-year battle with obesity and since about the age of ten she has gained and lost hundreds of pounds over and over again – and then she finally found *her own "weigh."*

In her previous attempts to lose weight Valerie's approach was always the same: exercise and regimented calorie restriction. It would work for a while and then eventually she'd creep back to old habits and before long the weight would creep back too.

When I asked Valerie what was different about the *last* time, her successful attempt, what she said surprised and delighted me. *I gave up on the idea of "perfect." When I started, I didn't try to brown-bag it every day, when before that I ate out all the time. I continued to go to my regular greasy spoon diner for lunch, but instead of the burger and fries, I ordered a burger patty without the bun, with a side of salad.*

*Instead of disallowing chocolate completely and forever, I allowed myself to have the occasional sugar-free chocolate. It didn't trigger cravings and out-of-control feelings like regular chocolate did, and I didn't feel deprived.*

*I learned to make low-calorie desserts instead of being really strict and punishing and not allowing myself any sweets at all.*

The bottom line for her was realizing that she has little control over her food choices when she regularly includes sugar and refined carbohydrates in her diet. As much as she enjoys them, she knows they don't work for her.

Once she cut those foods out her excessive hunger decreased, she stopped needing food before bed, cravings for junk food decreased, and her interest in healthier foods like lean protein and vegetables returned, plus she was satisfied with those choices.

Today, Valerie doesn't eat out as often as she used to. She packs her lunch almost every day but said *that evolved naturally over a longer period of time as I became more comfortable with my newer food choices.* As her weight loss progressed, the larger changes happened quite organically. It helped a lot that she allowed herself to develop those bigger lifestyle changes gradually instead of forcing herself to go big right out of the gate.

Valerie understands that eating right and exercise are necessary for overall health, but when it comes to weight management she says, *For me at least, healthy eating is the cornerstone of keeping the weight off. I can't exercise enough to exercise away the poor food choices.*

It's been almost seven years since she lost the weight and she admits that she still doesn't have it all figured out. She makes mistakes sometimes, but now she has enough tools, experience and belief in herself to get back on track quickly.

*I don't treat that knowledge lightly. It's not a free pass to make poor choices. I make mistakes just like anyone else, but I no longer live in fear of regaining all my weight again. If I consistently make the wrong choices I know it could come back quite easily, but I also know I can maintain this healthy lifestyle if I consistently make more right choices.*

Weight loss is hard work and that's not lost on Valerie. She, like so many people who have struggled with obesity, was told along the way that losing weight wouldn't magically change her life. The disagreeable boss, cranky husband, or crying child won't disappear with the weight.

Valerie agrees with that sentiment but also knows that her obesity was a far more draining aspect of her life than any of those things would ever have been. *Losing the weight, being able to let go of the sense of failure I felt every time I was unsuccessful in my attempts, regaining my health and energy, feeling happy in my body for the first time since I was a child − all of those things have improved the quality of my life dramatically. There is not a day that goes by that I don't feel like I won the lottery. My weight loss might not have been magical, but it sure feels like it to me.*

Valerie is another example of how small changes can bring forth big results. She worked hard, mined her past mistakes for clues on how to do it differently, and did *whatever it took* to find sustainable weight loss and a healthier more energetic life.

To learn more about Valerie and the work she does to coach people through their journey of weight loss, visit *www.findyourown-weigh.com*.

# ENERGY NOW!

## Nourishing Nibbles

- *At breakfast* have Canadian bacon at 90 calories for two slices instead of regular bacon at 250 calories for two slices. Have one slice of toast instead of two.
- *At lunch* order your greens with grilled (not crispy) chicken, shrimp, or salmon and low-fat dressing on the side.
- *At dinner* enjoy a great tasting turkey burger, not red meat. Have salad instead of fries for an even bigger caloric savings.
- *In baking* replace half of the fat in a recipe with applesauce. Per 1/2 cup, applesauce contains 90 calories, but butter or margarine contains a whopping 810 calories!
- Give up butter for a day. That tablespoon on your English muffin at breakfast, on your roll at lunch, and on your mashed potatoes at dinner adds up to at least 320 calories.
- At the coffee shop instead of your usual 16-ounce cafe mocha made with whole milk, have an 8-ounce one made with skim.
- Cut out two sugary drinks per day. These include alcoholic beverages, fruit juices, and any other drinks that have sugar in them.
- Cut that sandwich or wrap in half. Save the other half for another meal.
- Choose olive oil spray when cooking. Skip the butter, margarine, or liquid oils.
- Down-size your dishes. Pick a dinner plate or bowl that is smaller than your usual and you'll find you'll eat a lot less and still feel satisfied.
- Eat fewer meals in front of the TV. We eat more when we're distracted.
- Read nutrition labels. Get educated about the ingredients in your foods and the calories they pack and you'll make better decisions.
- Replace fattier sauces with vinegars, mustards, and lemon juice.

- Don't go too long without eating. You'll keep energy up, curb hunger and burn calories more efficiently if you eat small snacks every few hours.
- Plant a garden. Learn the wonders of growing your own food and experience the difference fresh makes.
- If you don't have yard space, investigate container gardening. You'd be amazed at what you can grow in small spaces.

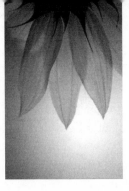

CHAPTER 7

# Hydration: *Water You Drinking?*

*Water is the driver of nature.*
—LEONARDO DA VINCI

A COUPLE of years ago I was convinced something was physically wrong with me. I was tired all the time. I had a tough time getting going in the morning, I would feel sluggish at times throughout the day – especially mid-afternoon between 2 and 4 p.m. – and even though I was getting good sleep, eating well most of the time and exercising regularly, I didn't feel healthy or energized. It didn't make sense.

Then as I was writing my *GOT TO IT* accountability journal I had an epiphany. The journal is designed to help you prioritize important self-care practices our busy lives cause us to skip, and includes daily checklists for keeping track of exercise, healthy eating efforts, and among other things *how much water you drink each day*. It was the only health-related item on my list that I wasn't as vigilant with and occurred to me that maybe I wasn't drinking enough water.

Could it be possible? I was skeptical because I always had water near me. I had a glass of water by my bedside all the time. I carried a water bottle with me throughout the day. I had a mug on my desk that was always full of water...and that was the problem – it was always *full* of water.

So I started to monitor my water intake. One check mark for every eight ounces I drank. What an eye-opener! I quickly learned that despite my best efforts to have water available to drink at all times, I was at best consuming two to three cups a day – about a third of the amount my body needed. Water, water, everywhere and not a drop I drank. Yikes! I was dehydrated!

I guess it shouldn't be surprising since an estimated 75 percent of North Americans are chronically dehydrated, but me? I'm a fitness professional, a Certified Exercise Physiologist. I have my Masters in Kinesiology, for crying out loud! But I guess if I was doing it and I know better, it helps explain why so few of us fail to consume enough healthy, energizing water. We need to be reminded of its numerous health benefits, and like any necessary task, we need to create a habit around its consumption.

## WATER *WORKS*

When you consider that the body is made up of 50 to 70 percent water it's no wonder it reacts badly when it is feeling parched. In fact, water is the second most important nutrient to the human body next to oxygen, and while you can go without food for months, you won't last more than a week without water.

Every system in your body depends on water. Consider the following health benefits of good hydration. If these truths don't get you guzzling more $H_2O$ every day, there may not be hope for your desert-like cells, but I think you'll find this interesting.

### Clear Thinking

Your brain is made up of 75 percent water, which is an essential element in neurological transmissions. You know those 70,000 thoughts you have each day? They're helped along by little zaps in your brain, and when you're dehydrated your grey-matter fire-power loses its oomph. Mild dehydration may be present with just a 1 to 2 percent drop in body water and can cause short-term memory problems and significant difficulties with concentration. If you drink more water you will remain mentally alert throughout the day. *That's using your smarts!*

## Fewer Headaches

That dull thud in your noggin isn't going to go away with a couple of aspirin or a jolt of caffeine. You need to drink more water! Since your brain's water content is so high, even slight dehydration can bring on a headache. So if you had a bit of alcohol last night or you haven't been drinking enough water in general, pay attention to your head. It's trying to tell you to drink more water.

## Temperature Control

On a hot day or during exercise your body cools itself by breaking out into a sweat. All of that liquid is pulled from the cells in your body as a protective mechanism against overheating and imminent system shutdown. It's why we need to drink so much more fluids in hot temperatures – preferably not all in the tall, frosty variety either. As long as you stay adequately topped up with water and other hydrating fluids your body will work to maintain a steady temperature of 37°C (98.6°F). This is vital for your health and safety because if your body temperature rises too high above that, you run the risk of not only dehydration, but heat exhaustion or heat stroke – both of which can be dangerous to your health, and in extreme cases, life threatening.

## Happy Digestive Function

Your digestive system needs a decent amount of water to aid in proper digestion of food. Since water is used by your body to help flush out toxins and waste products, when dehydrated you're more likely to experience constipation and stomach acid problems. And since chronic constipation has been linked with increased risk of colon cancer, it is even more appealing to stay hydrated and regular.

Additionally, if your body is adequately hydrated there will be enough fluid present in the digestive track to help distribute nutrients throughout the body. That means the foods you eat have a better chance of being utilized to their full nutritional capacity.

## Decreased Disease Risk

If you consider that every bodily function including brain function, immune system response, joint lubrication, digestive health and even cellular communication depend on the availability of adequate fluid in the body, it's not hard to understand how vital water is to our health.

Dehydration is at the root of many serious diseases, including asthma, kidney dysfunction, urinary tract infection, endocrine system and adrenal fatigue, high blood pressure and other cardiovascular problems, arthritis, ulcers and pancreatitis.

Research has shown that proper hydration may help to minimize chronic pain, such as that of rheumatoid arthritis, lower back pain, migraines, and colitis.

Some studies show hydration can decrease the risk of kidney stones and lower the risk of certain cancers by helping the body to flush out toxins.

Proper hydration can help asthmatics breathe more efficiently too. Given that lungs are nearly 90 percent water, dehydration interferes with how well they function, thereby increasing the likelihood of an asthma attack.

Drinking enough water can also lower your risks of a heart attack. A study published by the American Journal of Epidemiology found that men and women who drink more than five glasses of water a day were 54 percent and 41 percent, respectively, less likely to die from a heart attack during the study period than those who drank less than two glasses. More water intake means thinner blood that flows more easily through blood vessels in those at risk for heart attack.

*Have I convinced you yet?* Drink more water.

## Healthy Back and Joints

Adequate hydration has been shown to relieve back and joint pain for as many as 80 percent of sufferers. The disks between our vertebrae have two parts: an outer ring that is flexible and tough, and a gelatinous inner structure that is mostly water. As we travel upright through the day, gravity slowly squeezes the water out of the disks. It's why we're generally one-quarter to one-half inch shorter at the end of the day than we were at breakfast. While we sleep, the disks become rehydrated, drawing fluids from the cells around it. It's all good, unless you're dehydrated!

When there is not enough water available to fully hydrate the disk's center it shrinks and transfers more of its weight-bearing responsibilities to the less sturdy outer ring. Since the more rigid outer ring wasn't designed for these loads, the pressure eventually brings about pain, swelling, and even risk of a ruptured or herniated disk over time.

The moral of the story is: drink water and move regularly!

## That Healthy Glow

Water is one way to a better complexion. Proper hydration makes it possible for water to move through all the membranes of your body so that the largest organ in the body, your skin, is quenched with moisture. Skin texture softens, the natural aging process is slowed, wrinkles diminish and sagging skin tightens. When you've got water, who needs Botox?

## Wondrous Weight Management

As far as I'm concerned, water is one of the best tools to aid weight loss for four fabulous reasons:

1. When you start drinking more water, there's a good chance you'll drink fewer high-calorie drinks like soda, juice or even alcohol. If you consider that the average 355 ml (12 oz.) can of soda, orange juice or bottle of beer each have around 140 to 150 calories, you only need to forgo two of these beverages per day in favor of water, and in less than two weeks you'll be one pound lighter on the scale.

2. For over 30 percent of North Americans the thirst mechanism in the body is so weak that when we're feeling thirsty we mistake

that feeling for hunger and we eat instead of having water. Once you start drinking adequate amounts of $H_2O$ your thirst mechanism smartens up. It resets itself so that hunger is no longer confused with thirst, thereby eliminating consumption of those unnecessary calories. The obvious benefit: weight loss!

3. If you're trying to manage your weight through eating less, water can operate as a great appetite suppressant. Craving a bite when you know you don't need it? Drink a tall, cool glass of water. One glass of water shut down midnight hunger pangs for almost 100 percent of the dieters studied in a University of Washington study. It has no fat, no calories, no carbs and no sugar, and when your stomach is full of water, you'll feel less hungry.

4. Even mild dehydration will slow down your metabolism by as much as 3 percent. This means your body will burn calories more slowly than it should and you run the risk of storing extra calories as fat.

Drink more water and burn, baby, burn!

## More Energy

Lack of water is the #1 trigger of daytime fatigue. Dehydration can very quickly sap your energy and make you feel tired. Even mild dehydration of as little as 1 or 2 percent of your body weight can lead to fatigue, muscle weakness, dizziness and other symptoms – all of which will impact your productivity and enthusiasm for what is going on around you.

Imagine how that fatigue will affect your eagerness for getting active. Since physical fitness is a sure-fire energizer, double your efforts by drinking energizing water so you have energy for energizing exercise. Say that six times fast!

The hydration health benefits I've listed above should be enough to convince you that it's essential to drink plenty of water, all day, every day, but what does that really mean?

*So how do I know if I'm dehydrated?* Signs of dehydration aren't always obvious. You probably have days when you rush around on little or no sleep, maybe you had a few drinks last night, perhaps your muscles are tired from carrying those boxes, or it could be that you don't know what energetic and healthy feels like, so this is normal for you. Uh oh! We need to do something about this! Symptoms of dehydration can include:

- Mild to excessive thirst
- Fatigue
- Headache
- Dry mouth
- Little or no urination
- Muscle weakness
- Dizziness
- Lightheadedness

If you're experiencing any or all of these symptoms on a regular basis, get yourself to a water fountain ASAP! There is a good chance you're dehydrated and it's time to start bathing your body cells in the wonderful water they're screaming for.

On a slightly more serious note, it's important to mention that the above symptoms can also be signs of other more critical ailments. You know your body better than anyone else. If you think you're dehydrated, drink up and see if you start to feel better. If you have doubts about your health, it's always good to consult with a doctor or medical professional to be sure.

## EXERCISE AND FLUID REPLACEMENT

If you are active – especially in warmer climates – it's essential that you increase your water intake to help with water lost as sweat. In one hour of exercise your body can lose as much as a liter of water, depending on the air temperature and the intensity of your workout.

It's a good idea to drink more fluids leading up to your workout, and then sip every fifteen minutes or so during your workout so you stay topped up. To ensure you properly replace lost fluids at the end of an intense workout, try this method. Weigh yourself at the beginning and end of your workout. For every pound of weight you are down (this weight loss will be predominantly water weight), make sure you drink 16 to 24 oz (2 to 3 cups) of water to rehydrate.

*All right, but how much water should I drink every day?*

Believe it or not, there isn't a recommended water intake that fits everyone. Most information about water consumption suggests you drink eight 8-ounce glasses of water every day (2 litres) but few can cite where that information originated. It's not a bad guideline though. Sip early and sip often. Your body will tell you when it is better hydrated – if only by the number of trips you need to take to the restroom!

## CHECKS AND BALANCES

Here are three things you can monitor to make sure you continue to stay hydrated every day.

### Am I thirsty?

Well, this one is an obvious one, but if you're thirsty I don't want you to ignore it anymore. If you're feeling thirsty, it's too late. You're already heading toward dehydration, so it's situation critical to top up on those hydrating fluids.

### What color is my pee?

Yeah, you read correctly. If you want to stay hydrated you need to become a bowl watcher. Once you're done going #1 look at the color of your pee. If it's a dark yellow color and has a strong odor, you haven't been drinking enough water. If you've been drinking enough water your urine will be light yellow or clear in color. Nice work!

Pay attention to volume as well. If you do not produce much

urine throughout the day and it is dark in color, you likely need more fluids.

### How am I feeling?

Remember my confession at the start of this chapter? I was feeling tired and unfocused despite decent rest and nutrition. If you feel light-headed and tired, or unable to concentrate, or are experiencing frequent headaches, pay attention! These could be signs that you're dehydrated.

☑    8 glasses per day and you're on your way.

☑    Add on when you're active.

☑    Pay attention to the signs.

Yes, I do think water is best, but there are other ways to healthfully hydrate too. Try to avoid beverages with too much sugar or caffeine. Sugar has calories and caffeine is a diuretic. I talk about each in more detail below. Consider herbal teas, diluted juices, or flavored water as alternatives to the plain stuff. ENERGY NOW! at the end of this chapter lists *dozens* of ideas for faithfully keeping those fluids flowing.

## LESS SODAS, JUICES, AND SUGARY DRINKS

*I really hate the taste of water.* You would be amazed how often I hear this statement from people. I guess it confuses me since water is essentially tasteless and odorless. Maybe the more accurate admission is that water is boring. Fair enough. If you're not a water drinker you can still hydrate by drinking other beverages, but I want to share a few thoughts with you and hopefully steer you back to the water cooler – plain and simple.

We often tell ourselves juice is okay. *It has vitamins and nutrients that are good for me!* Yes, 100 percent pure juice has vitamins and nutrients that are good for you, but it also contains a lot of sugar. Just a single glass of 100 percent juice is 150 calories and contains about seven teaspoons of sugar. Ouch! So not only are you cutting into your daily calorie allotment *big time*, but you're adding unnecessary sugar to your diet. The same is true for sodas and other sugary drinks like sports beverages or energy drinks.

If you currently drink juice or soda in lieu of water you'd need to consume a fair bit to ensure decent hydration. If each soda or juice serving is a minimum of 150 calories, then your daily juice or soda intake will add up quickly. In Chapter 6 I suggest that calorie counting is not the best way to establish a healthy relationship with food, but if you're attempting to manage your weight and live more energetically, you can achieve that easily by watching your liquid calories.

Let's say you decided to cut out just one sugary beverage per day. At 150 calories a pop, in seven days you will have saved 1050 calories. With that one little change you'll eliminate about 50 teaspoons (about 1 cup) of energy-sapping sugar and lose one pound in about three weeks.

Imagine if you were to replace all your sugary beverages with water? Even three sugary drinks per day at 150 calories each total 450 calories. With those savings you'll be down a pound in seven days.

If weight management isn't on your mind then consider how all of that sugar is gumming up your system. Too much sugar will not only affect weight gain and tooth decay, but over time it could contribute to other health problems, like insulin resistance. Sugar can cause an increase of insulin in the blood. Insulin resistance is when your body cells have been flooded with insulin for so long that they lose their sensitivity to it. Insulin is the hormone that allows cells to use glucose (or sugar) for energy and if cells are resistant to insulin your body must produce more of it to be effective. The end result is diabetes.

A 2010 study published in the *Journal of the American Medical Association* suggests that too much sugar in the diet can also contribute to heart disease in much the same way as too much fat. It found that people who consumed more added sugar were more likely to have higher risk factors for heart disease, such as higher triglycerides and lower levels of protective high-density lipoprotein or HDL cholesterol.

So there you go. Is all that sugar really worth it? Consider the pros and cons. Find balance in your fluid consumption. If you choose a sugar-sweetened beverage, go for the small size once or twice a day. Opt instead for healthy, low-calorie beverages; try some of the ideas at the end of this chapter; or embrace good, simple, refreshing water as your hydrating beverage of choice.

## CHARGE!

Boy oh BOY. If you do nothing else in your effort to get more energy, I encourage you to take the advice in this chapter. Drink more water. This week drink one more glass than you normally do and replace one sugary drink with another glass.

Maybe you'll be running to the washroom more often but you can just count that as a bit more exercise. Try at least one of the ENERGY NOW tips below every day this week and begin to feel the benefits of heavenly hydration on your health and energy now!

### WHATEVER IT TAKES

Bob – a participant in one of my workshops – has a waterful weight loss story worth sharing. He was a reasonably healthy man who exercised regularly and ate mostly healthfully but he had a vice that was impacting his weight. He had a big, bad soda habit.

Six months earlier Bob had started a new job that necessitated an early start and long days. To keep his energy up he started drinking cola – four or five 18-ounce (533ml) bottles every day. His excuse was that he didn't like coffee.

He bought flats of soda and had bottles stashed in his car, and in the fridge at work and home.

At 218 calories a bottle, the sodas accounted for over 1000 extra calories every day that his body didn't need. Those calories went straight to Bob's belly. He wanted to lose about twenty-five pounds.

On his forty-seventh birthday Bob's present to himself was to give up cola cold turkey. At first he suffered from sugar withdrawal and admitted to the occasional diet cola when he needed a caffeine jolt, but other than that he drank water.

He was astonished by how quickly he saw results. In the first week alone Bob lost three pounds, noticing that the absence of sugary cola in his diet decreased cravings for other sweets as well.

Not only that, but by drinking water instead of soda he had *more* energy, not less. The energy he gained from the sugary, caffeine-rich sodas was often short-lived and left him jittery. Water seemed to help him stay alert and energized all through the day.

The hydrating benefits of water were so apparent that his work day and his workouts gained energy-driven momentum and added to his results.

In one month Bob lost fourteen pounds – more than half of his goal weight – simply by replacing soda with water and riding the energy wave to an even healthier lifestyle.

Bob also figures he's saved hundreds of dollars every month not buying soda. If you're a soda drinker, try Bob's waterful *whatever it takes* weight loss method.

## ENERGY NOW!

### Make Hydration a Habit

- Spice up plain old water by adding fresh mint leaves. Mmmm, refreshing!
- Instead of setting down an empty glass, refill it with water and keep sipping.
- Every time you pass a water cooler stop and take a sip.
- If you're feeling hungry and you've eaten recently, drink a cold glass of water, and wait a minute or two. You could just be dehydrated!
- Make your water more interesting by adding a squeeze of lemon or lime.
- Add ice cubes to your water – this helps to burn calories when your body brings the water temperature up.
- Dilute your juice (apple, grape, or orange) with water. It's usually too sweet anyway! More hydration with less calories!

- Make it a morning ritual. Start your day by drinking one or two glasses of water. Start early, feel better, set the trend for the day.

- Eat water-rich foods like watermelon (92 percent water by weight) for a refreshing, hydrating break from sipping. Just be sure to include the calories in your daily plan.

- Have a big glass of water at every transitional point of the day: when you first get up, before you leave the house, when you sit down to work, when you go to lunch…

- Get a glass you love. My water mug says "Today is the start of a new journey" and I'm inspired to sip from it every time I look at it.

- After each trip to the restroom, drink some water to replenish your system.

- Okay, I know it's less fun, but every now and then when you're out for cocktails ask yourself "Do I really want this?" At some social functions choose sparkling soda instead.

- Drink water or diet drinks instead of high-calorie, sugar-sweetened drinks.

- Instead of spending a fortune on bottled water, save your money and the environment and invest in a filter for your home faucet. Or get a portable Brita. Make tap water taste like bottled, at a fraction of the price.

- Have a glass of water with your meal, especially when you're drinking alcohol.

- Take a bottle of water with you on your walks.

- Carry a bottle you like! Mine is a traditional plastic Nalgene that I've covered in stickers. I bought an easy-sip mouth piece so it doesn't spill when I'm sipping on the go.

- Freeze little bits of peeled lemons, limes, and oranges and use them in place of ice cubes - it's refreshing and helps get in a serving of fruit.

- While at work, fill a big glass with ice and keep filling it up from the office water cooler.

- At home always keep a glass of water handy while watching TV, doing laundry, making dinner or surfing the net.

- Replace your coffee or tea with a cup of hot water and a drop of honey.

- Keep water cold. Some find it tastes better and your body will burn some calories bringing it to body temperature.

- Room temperature water is better if you're dehydrated. Your body absorbs it more quickly.

- Drink through a straw and you'll take bigger gulps and drink much more.

- Build up your $H_2O$ levels. Start with one or two glasses first thing in the morning and add on.

- Carry a small refillable water bottle at all times and drink while you wait...standing in line, sitting in traffic, or even waiting for the elevator.

- Track it. Once I started keeping track of my water intake it went up. One check mark for every glass consumed ☑ .

- Visualize your healthy, glowing skin.

- "I have to pee every ten minutes." As you run off to the restroom yet again, remind yourself of the extra exercise you're getting as you do!

- Add water to your daily skincare regimen. Drink, cleanse, moisturize, then drink again.

- Remember that the more water you drink, the less hungry you will feel and the less likely you will be to snack.

- Water by itself doesn't contain any calories or fat, and has so many health benefits hidden in its plainness!

- Don't allow yourself a diet soda or another coffee until you've had two to four glasses of water.

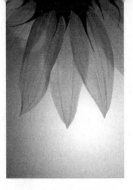

CHAPTER 8

# Sleep:
# The Quest for Rest
# and Relaxation

*Sleep is the golden chain that ties health and our bodies together.*
—Thomas Dekker

W HEN I was personal training full time I was up before
dawn most days of the week to meet my clients before
they headed to work. Despite my early mornings I
would stay up late watching television or hanging out with friends.
I survived on five or six hours and I was tired all the time, only I
didn't realize to what extent.

My body was so used to running on empty that I thought
this was normal. My work days began at 5:30 a.m. and often stretched
into the dinner hour. Before long my coping skills began to decline
and I eventually fell into a state of burnout that had me rethinking
my work schedule. I needed to prioritize rest and recovery, pronto!

# Zzzzzzz's PLEASE!

It's surprising to me how frequently I hear people oppose the idea that sleep is necessary. I've listened to dozens of full-grown, seemingly intelligent adults tell me they can get by on much less sleep than the average person, or that they have *way* too much to do to warrant getting to bed at a decent hour.

Sure they're tired they tell me in one breath, but they don't have a choice I hear in the next. *Is there a place around here I can grab a coffee?* And by the way, I often wonder *why would you just want to get by?*

Perhaps you gave up the idea of restorative, health-giving zzz's when false energy became abundantly available in the form of pills, elixirs and energy beverages? After all, caffeine is not illegal, and *man* those energy drinks can pack a punch!

Maybe you really want to sleep better and longer but you're trapped in the daily grind of too much to do and not enough time to do it? I've had entire audiences tell me that if they were given extra time in the day to do whatever they pleased, they'd choose to sleep.

It could be that you need ideas and tactics to prepare for sleep and stage your bedroom for optimal sleep.

Or perhaps you've been wandering around in a sleep-deprived state for so long now that you've forgotten what it feels like to wake up without your alarm clock, feeling refreshed, alert and keen to get on with the day? If you identify with any of these scenarios, then read on, my groggy friend.

## The Quest for Rest

I'm not certain when sleep became a luxury, but it seems to be something that many of us top up on once the weekend arrives, or on the next vacation. I'm here to tell you that's not how it works.

Rest is not something that can be gained through infrequent overdoses. It's a daily requirement alongside energy-producing exercise and healthy eating. Why fight it?

It reminds me of my nieces and nephews when they were young. They would regularly fight with their parents around bedtime, insisting through droopy eyelids and stifled yawns that they weren't tired yet. Fatigue had made them irrational and at four and five years of age caffeine and energy drinks were out of the question so they would lose the battle and be carted off to bed. But not you.

You'll fight it until the last possible moment, fitting in more housework, another load of laundry, endless emails and internet surfing or mindless television until you drift into a fitful sleep on the sofa. You call that restoration?

## BENEFITS OF SLEEP

If you're sleep-deprived, make no mistake, it will eventually impact every aspect of your daily life. Sleep has many benefits. It provides energy and helps us feel better, but there's a lot more to it than that.

The Division of Sleep Medicine at Harvard Medical School has done a great deal of research on the effects of sleep. Not surprisingly, these studies have shown time and again that sleep plays a key role in promoting physical health, longevity, and emotional wellbeing.

It's true, isn't it? After a good night's sleep you just feel better. Thoughts are clearer, emotions less fragile, and contentment higher.

While many benefits of sleep are obvious, you may be interested to learn some of the lesser known advantages of quality slumber.

### Repair Your Body

Throughout the day your body is beat down through physical stress as well as UV rays, environmental pollutants and even germs. While you sleep your body produces more protein – the building block for cells – which helps repair your body and boost your immune system. Lack of sleep will eventually take its toll through more frequent illness and injury.

### Perk Up Your Mood

Inadequate sleep impacts your judgment, increases agitation and muddies your mood. Most of us can navigate the occasional sleep-lessness-induced grumpy spell, but you want to avoid chronic sleep deficiency, which can lead to mood disorders like anxiety or depression.

## Improve Your Memory

Fatigue has a negative impact on concentration and memory. The more tired you get, the more difficulty you will have in recalling incidents, lessons, faces and facts. The good news is that while you sleep the filing cabinets in your brain have time to get organized, imprint the day's new knowledge and information, and improve your memory. If you often forget the details it will pay to simply *sleep on it.*

## Boost Your Energy

After a good night's sleep who doesn't feel more energized and alert? You can use that energy to boost your energy. Take your invigorated body outdoors. Engage with your surroundings and do active things. You'll sleep better again that night and gain even more energy.

## Reduce Your Stress

Sleep deprivation is a form of stress that will prompt the release of stress hormones in the body, which not only increase your blood pressure, but also increase risk of gastric distress and ulcers.

Yes, stress can impact your ability to sleep, so practice breathing techniques, stretching or meditation to help you relax before bed.

## Improve Your Health

Chronic sleep deprivation can lead to serious medical conditions such as diabetes, heart disease, hypertension, obesity and even premature death. Many of the body's mechanisms against these diseases are enhanced while we sleep. The way I see it, you can't afford not to.

## Manage Your Weight

Research suggests that those who get less than seven hours of sleep per night are more likely to be overweight. It seems that when your body is sleep-deprived, normal hormone balance is disrupted and your appetite increases. Unfortunately, the foods your body craves in these instances are usually high-fat, carbohydrate-loaded comfort foods, *not* healthy fruits and vegetables.

If you're hanging on to a few stubborn pounds, then add quality sleep into your weight management routine. You can't lose. Well actually, you can!

## Live Longer

Is there a better reason to make quality sleep a priority? Studies show that people who regularly get an appropriate amount of sleep live longer, healthier lives than those who don't. I guess the obvious question then is...

# How Much Is Enough?

I wish this was an easy question to answer. Most experts agree that when it comes to quantifying ideal amounts of sleep there is no magic number. Sleep needs will vary by age, and are as individual as a fingerprint.

While a very small percentage of the population will be able to function on less sleep, most adults will function best with somewhere between seven to nine hours per night. But it's not that simple.

National Sleep Foundation research suggests that quality sleep is a function of two factors: your basal sleep needs, which is the amount of sleep your body requires to function optimally, and your sleep debt, or the amount of sleep you lose to poor sleep, illness or other factors. Put simply, the quantity and quality of your sleep.

It's not enough to log a consistent seven hours per night if your sleep quality is poor or if your body actually needs more. To ensure optimal zzz's for outstanding energy do some sleep research of your own to determine your specific needs.

## Sleep 101

The first step in your sleep evaluation is to pay attention to how you feel as you wake up and go through your day. If you've had enough sleep you should feel energetic and awake the entire work day, and still have energy to spare for family and after work activities. That would be nice, wouldn't it?

However, if you're like most busy people you probably wake up lacking energy or you feel drained before the day is out. To truly feel your best you need to get more rest.

Begin by scheduling an extra half hour or more of sleep each night. Keep a sleep diary and record your bedtime, total hours you sleep and how you feel upon waking. Before long you'll begin to see a pattern and be able to hone in on your magic number. Once you have that number then make it your goal to schedule that amount of sleep every night.

I know it's not always that simple. Many people allow enough time for sleep but then find themselves tossing and turning through the night. Maybe you can't fall asleep, or you fall asleep easily but have trouble staying asleep? I don't know if there is anything more frustrating.

Regardless of your circumstances I'm hoping by now you understand the importance of sleep for restoration, everyday energy, and long-term health, and are willing to explore your sleep options. Let's look at two aspects of healthy sleep: the routine or rituals that will help you sleep better, and your sleep environment.

## SLEEP ROUTINE

How can you expect to fall into blissful sleep if you race through a hectic day and then over-stimulate your mind with high-intensity television, blast your brain cells with internet information overload, or keep working right up until lights out?

And your body won't wind down well if you feed it unhealthy snacks or too much food or alcohol right before bed.

If you want to ensure restorative sleep, the first step revolves around your sleep routine. Your goal is to create an environment in the hours before bedtime that will allow your mind and body to ease into a sleep receptive state.

### Unwind Early

If you know you need to get to bed by 10 p.m. it won't do your sleep efforts any good to be moving at high speed until 9:55. Shut down the television, computer, video games or other high-stimulus activities at least thirty, and ideally sixty, minutes before sleep. Allow your mind to shift gears from work mode to sleep mode.

## Eat, Drink and Be Healthy

Your body is a great big machine that stays fired up as long as you give it food and drink to metabolize. Avoid big meals at night. Eat dinner earlier and avoid heavy, fatty foods or any food you know could bother you later.

To get a good night's sleep limit your alcohol intake. It may help you fall asleep faster but it reduces the quality of your sleep and you'll likely wake up at 2:30 a.m. with a dry mouth and headache.

Cut down on caffeine. I can't have caffeine any time after 2 p.m. if I hope to sleep well at night. Some people can have sleep problems from caffeine they drank ten hours ago! Why not switch to water or herbal tea after lunch?

Hydrate, but not too late. If you drink lots of tea, juice or water into the evening there's a good chance you'll be up in the middle of the night for a bathroom break.

There are hundreds of reasons to quit smoking, and sleep trouble is one of them. That nasty nicotine is a stimulant that will keep you awake longer and since you may experience nicotine withdrawal through the night it will affect your sleep. Besides, smoking is no way to start your day.

## Relax with a Ritual

If you find it difficult to shut off the stress of the day, try slowing down with a bedtime routine that promotes relaxation. Take a hot bath or sip on a warm cup of chamomile tea. Do some slow stretches or deep breathing. Listen to some calming music or meditate. Make simple plans for the next day. Read or do a favorite hobby. Lower the lights to induce production of melatonin, the hormone that helps you fall, and stay, asleep. Every small effort you make in the direction of calm will add quality to your sleepy time.

## Set a Sleep Schedule

Yes, I know you're an adult and should be allowed to stay up as long as you like, but unless you are free to sleep in endlessly that behavior will catch up with your energy levels if it hasn't already.

You've got a good idea how many hours of sleep your body really needs to work at its best. Why not see how it actually makes you feel?

Ideally you'll choose the same bedtime every night so your body gets into a routine. Get to bed early enough that you consistently get enough rest and before long you'll be waking up refreshed and energized *before* your alarm clock.

## To Nap or Not to Nap

Be cautious about napping during the day. It can be a great way to recharge or catch up on sleep but if you nap too late in the day you may have trouble sleeping at night. If a nap is necessary, keep it to less than thirty minutes in the early afternoon.

If your evening television vigil often ends with you snoring on the sofa, beware! Fight the urge to nod off. If it's near bedtime go to bed. If it's still early get up and do something mildly reviving.

Pack your workout gear and make your healthy lunch for tomorrow, call your mom, put away the dishes. That late night nap will cut the edge off your fatigue just enough to leave you staring at the ceiling at bedtime.

## Clear Your Head

A quick journaling session at the end of the day is a great way to clear your head of worrying thoughts or lingering to-do's. Before lights out, allow yourself five minutes to write down all your stressors: a work problem, a conflict with someone, a financial worry – and maybe even one or two steps you can take toward resolving the stress.

Before you put the journal away write down at least three things you are grateful for. Put your stress to rest so you can have rest success.

## Use Good Scents

Aromatherapy oils like chamomile, juniper, lavender, marjoram, rose and sandalwood all have a sedative effect when inhaled.

Rub a wee bit on the insides of your wrists or on your temples and breathe in the relaxing fragrance as you drift into dreamland.

## Sleep Environment

Okay, so you created a routine and have been sticking to it faithfully, and still quality sleep eludes you. The next step then is to optimize your sleep environment.

### Get a Good Bed

Did you know that we spend about one-third of our lives in bed? If you want those hours to be comfortable and restful it's essential that you invest in a mattress suited to your body and its biomechanical needs.

Comfort is key. If you can't seem to find a comfortable position on your bed no matter how tired you are or which way you lie, you probably have the wrong mattress.

When shopping for beds sit and lie down on each one for several minutes at a time. Just don't shop for them when you're tired, because every bed is bound to feel good.

### Better Bedding

You'll improve your sleep with soft, comfortable bedding that will allow for proper temperature control. Sheets with a higher thread count made from 100 percent cotton or silk will feel more luxurious than synthetic fabrics like polyester.

Purchase the right pillow for your personal comfort preference and sleep style. Try several out before you buy. It's a worthwhile investment in your alignment and comfort.

### Go to the Dark Side

To ensure the best sleep possible make your bedroom a low-light zone. Your body won't produce melatonin – the sleep hormone – unless it experiences darkness.

At bedtime keep your room dimly lit. Make sure window coverings block out all outside light, especially during the long daylight hours of summer. Use a comfortable eye mask if necessary. And keep the television out of the bedroom. Not only does your TV emit a lot of melatonin-busting light, but it keeps your senses stimulated and less capable of deep restful sleep.

## Keep Your Cool

Your body temperature rises as you sleep. If you begin your slumber in a warm room you're likely to overheat and wake yourself up as you kick free of your bedding. Keep your bedroom temperature around 65° F or 18° C and allow for adequate ventilation.

## PJ Preference

Whether you wear a satin negligee or flannel jammies, make sure your PJ of preference keeps you warm and comfortable throughout the night. If you wear your birthday suit to bed then ensure that your bedding fulfills that role.

Choose pyjamas that won't bind or wrap around you as you sleep. Cotton may be crisp but silk will keep you cool in summer and warm in winter. The perfect PJ will add quality to your sleep.

## Silence Please

You'll have difficulty falling asleep and staying asleep if your sleep environment is plagued by unpredictable noises. Close your bedroom door to block out furnace noises or family members.

If your bedmate snores or mumbles in their sleep, or you can't block out traffic or other outdoor noises, try sleeping with ear plugs.

Ear plugs rated at 33 decibels will block out most distracting noises and you'll still be able to hear the smoke detector if it goes off.

Yes, they may fall out while you sleep but they'll stay in long enough for you to get into deeper sleep that will block out some of the noises around you.

## White Noise Works

If the idea of sticking rubber bits in your ears makes you shudder, try the soothing sound of crickets or ocean waves instead.

The noises that keep us awake usually vary in tempo and volume. You can often drown out these noises with the steady rhythm of a white noise machine. The steady hum of a fan will have the same benefit and cool your room at the same time.

## Breathe Easy

Even though you're an adult I'm going to say this to you one more time. Clean your room. A bedroom full of dust and musty air is difficult to sleep in.

Change the bed sheets at least once a week. At the same time dust the furniture and sweep the floors – even under the bed; and especially if you have pets. Open the windows to let in fresh air. If there are no windows in your room a plant or two will improve air quality and add to your relaxing sleep environment.

We have an air filter in our room that we turn on during the day to remove dust and dander from the air before bed. A humidifier is also a good idea if your room is dry.

## Sleep and Sex

There really are only two things that should happen in your bedroom. Sleep and sex. If you're not experiencing sex – and even if you are – it's not a good idea to replace that option with television, ever.

You may argue that you're able to fall asleep to the flickering light of the television screen, the noises and disturbing late night TV content but I really want you to rethink this.

I guarantee you're impacting the quality of your sleep either because it's not as deep as it could be or because you're jolted out of sleep from some 3:00 a.m. cop show shoot out.

You're also sending a message to your brain that the bed is not just a place for sleep and leisure it's also for wide-awake-sit-and-stare-into-space television. How is that going to help your sleep habits?

The television may also be getting in the way of your intimate relationship and since sex helps you sleep *and* provides exercise I'm all for promoting a healthy sex life.

Dr. Trina Read, sex and relationship expert and author of *Till Sex Do Us Part*, agrees. *If you want a good sex life, get the TV out of your bedroom!*

In fact she says it's not just the TV. The bedroom needs to be an electronic-free zone: no TV, IPods, computer, Blackberry or latest tech gizmo. They are simply distractions and the more you engage in the technology the more you disengage from your partner.

A partnership can successfully survive without sex but it can't survive without intimacy. It is intimacy, not sex, that is the glue that holds a couple together through thick and thin. It also allows them to experience deeper emotions while having sex.

Couples need to create a space where intimacy and closeness can thrive and that means no distractions. A healthy and happy partnership will last only so long if it's being neglected.

And here's another thought. Television in the bedroom reduces the quality of your sleep so you're tired all the time, and when you're tired you'll likely be less interested in sex. Get it out of there!

Chronic sleep deprivation can have long-term effects on your health. Some sleep problems can't be solved by routine and environment alone. If you think you suffer from insomnia, sleep apnea, or any other sleep disorder, then see a sleep specialist. They'll assess your situation and advise you on methods and treatments for regaining quality sleep.

## Sleepless Solutions

If you find yourself unable to fall asleep, or you are staring at the ceiling at 3:00 a.m. unable to fall back to sleep, let go of dread. Follow these tips instead.

*Don't think so much about it.* In order to regain sleep you need to cue your body for sleep. Take a few deep breaths of air and allow your body to relax into a normal sleep position.

Try not to stress about the sleep you're not getting and desperately need. That will only keep you awake. When I have difficulty sleeping I repeat two words in my mind as I breathe.

As I breathe in slowly I think *calm* and as I breathe out I think *sleep.* Calm...sleep...calm...sleep...calm...zzzzz.

*Focus first on relaxation.* Willing yourself back to sleep is akin to using the buzz of the alarm clock as a relaxation tool. It won't work.

Focus first on relaxation and let it lead naturally to sleep. Try visualizing a relaxing environment, focus on slow deep breathing, or meditate with soothing words like the ones I mention above.

Relaxation may not be a true replacement for sleep but it will still keep you on the path to rest and recovery.

*Get out of bed.* If sleep eludes you for a period of time longer than twenty minutes, get out of bed and do a quiet activity like reading or knitting. Keep the lights low so you stay in a sleep-receptive state. If hunger pangs are part of the problem, have a light snack. A few spoonfuls of yogurt or a small piece of cheese can provide satiety without stimulating your system into wakefulness.

*Write down your thoughts.* If you wake up midway through the night with a great idea that is keeping you awake, write it down so your brain can quit worrying that you'll forget it. Expand on the idea the next day when energy and productivity are higher.

If you wake up wracked with worry or anxiety about something, write it down and give yourself permission to deal with it in daylight, when coping mechanisms are optimized.

## Daytime Restoration Exploration

Rest and relaxation isn't just for bedtime anymore. As you rush busily through your day think of ways that you can slow down and catch a breath. Small breathing breaks throughout the day will do wonders to moderate your stress levels and add a little restoration to an otherwise crazy day.

- Take your coffee breaks at work. Take a walk or just sit and breathe.
- Get outside at least once per day. Breathe in the fresh air.
- Eat your lunch away from your desk. Sit and savor.
- Put on your headphones and listen to soothing music for five minutes.
- Explore relaxation techniques that you can do on the go.
- Engage in a twenty-second mini-meditation. Close your eyes and breathe to the bottom of your lungs for four slow, calming breaths.
- Practice speaking more slowly. You'll feel yourself slow down with it.
- On your way home from work decompress with music or go get some exercise.

So there you go – dozens of ideas to help you improve the quality of your sleep. The *rest* is up to you. If you're always tired and you know you need more sleep, then it's time to make it a priority.

You schedule time for work and other commitments so why wouldn't you schedule in your sleep commitments?

From this day on promise yourself that you won't cut back on sleep in the quest to conquer your to-do list. I'm quite certain that if you make sleep a priority the energy you gain will make you more productive during the day anyway. It will all get done. Now, go to bed!

## CHARGE!

If you're chronically sleep-deprived it can be very difficult to catch up on those energy-giving zzzzz's. Why not schedule a sleep vacation?

Try this on your next two-week holiday or pick a couple of weeks in your schedule when you have some flexibility.

Go to bed at the same time every night and let yourself sleep until you naturally wake up. Don't you dare turn on that alarm clock.

This routine will reset your sleep debt and you'll tune in to a sleep schedule that's ideal for you.

### WHATEVER IT TAKES

Melinda, one of my always-tired clients, laughed at me when I suggested a sleep vacation. *What do you suggest that I do with my children? Let the dog feed and clothe them?*

She had a good point. With two small kids at home the sleep schedule wasn't always hers to set. Perhaps a two-week sleep vacation was unrealistic for her, but it didn't change the fact that she really needed sleep.

Melinda and I talked about creative ways she could increase the quality and quantity of her sleep.

- She began by asking her parents to take the kids for a weekend and she used that time to rest, relax and catch up on sleep.

- The next week she purchased a wake-up clock for the kid's room. She set the sunshine to 7:15 a.m. and explained to her four-year-old that when the sun shone on the clock it was okay to get up... but not before. If they woke up earlier he and his two-and-a-half-year-old sister would chatter with each other until sunshine time.★

- As a stay-at-home mom she decided that when she needed to, she'd nap when her kids did. Laundry could wait.

- She started going to bed an hour earlier most nights and implemented some of the sleep techniques I write about in this chapter.

- On Saturdays she asked her husband to make breakfast for the kids so she could sleep a little longer.

The sleep steps Melinda made were indeed small ones, but after two weeks of making sleep a higher priority she admitted that she felt more alert and less stressed.

What will you do to improve the quality and quantity of sleep you're getting? It's a necessary investment in your health, happiness and energy. Do whatever it takes.

★*A wake-up clock is a fabulous invention for any parent who has early-riser kids. You set the clock for the time you want your kids to stay in bed until. When that time comes, the display will show a wake-up scene which is the indicator for your child that it's now all right to get out of bed.* How great is that?

---

## ENERGY NOW!

### Sleep Tight

- Record your favorite late night show and go to bed an hour earlier tonight.

- No more caffeinated beverages after 1 p.m.

- Walk away from TV an hour before bed.

- Oh go on, save the laundry for another day. Take that nap. You know you want to.
- Meditate for five minutes before you hit the sack.
- Or just breathe deeply and slowly. Same diff.
- Exchange massages with your partner. If you're tired it will soothe you into restful sleep.
- Sip on chamomile tea.
- Avoid high-protein and fatty snacks within two hours of bedtime. They take longer to digest.
- Exercise during the day will help you sleep better at night. Walk on!
- Turn off the computer and read before bed instead.
- A nice warm bath or shower is a great way to relax and unwind before sleepy time.
- If you must have a night cap, keep it to just one. Too much alcohol disrupts the sleep cycle.
- There are only two activities that should take place in the bedroom. TV isn't one of them.
- Clean your room! You'll sleep better if your sheets are clean and your space is dust-free.
- Quit smoking please. It's the wrong kind of stimulant for the bedroom.
- Luxuriate in great pyjamas.
- Keep your room cool and dark to promote deep, comfortable sleep.

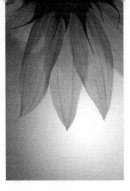

CHAPTER 9

# Stress Less for Success

*There is more to life than increasing its speed.*
—MOHANDAS K. GANDHI

I F you had less stress how would your life be different? How would you feel? What would you do with all of your time and energy?

These are important questions to ponder on the path to less stress, but like most busy people you likely just accept stress as an interminable, inevitable part of life.

*It has always been here and always will. So I just deal with it.*

I hear that from a lot of busy people who tell me they don't have time to do what's necessary to manage their stress, so they just deal with it until the negative effects of stress catch up and drag them down.

Stress is an insidious energy sucker. From a physical standpoint it will rob you of health and vitality in the short term, and left unchecked will bring on weight gain, life-threatening illness and even death.

From a mental and emotional point of view stress impacts concentration, mood, and memory function. It affects decision making, creativity and productivity day to day.

## Stress Express

Despite these truths, stress is an inevitable and sometimes necessary part of life. Stress is how your body responds to danger – an imminent attack or a house fire, for instance. The chemical reactions that take place during stressful situations prepare your body to fight the enemy or get out fast so life can get back to normal.

These days we're not always fighting the big fight though, are we? In today's busy world stress seems to come at us from all angles and varying low-level amounts.

Traffic, high work load, endless emails and phone calls, financial stress, aging parents, young kids and work worry flood us with endless little hits of stress that the body finds difficult to recover from.

In order to understand the drain of modern-day or chronic stress it might first help to understand how normal or acute stress impacts the body.

In his pivotal research, stress pioneer Hans Selye identified three stages of stress response: how your body reacts to, combats, and recovers from stress.

### Alarm, Recuperation, Relaxation

The first stage of the stress response is the *alarm* stage, when your body meets with a stressful event. You may have heard the term *fight or flight* associated with stress at this stage.

Whether you are fleeing a charging grizzly or fighting heavy traffic, your body is told to prepare for action.

It releases adrenalin and another fight-or-flight hormone called *cortisol,* and your body kicks into gear.

Blood pressure and heart rate increase, pupils dilate, blood is redirected to the working muscles, blood sugar increases, gastric secretions increase, blood coagulates more rapidly – all to prepare you for battle.

When danger is real (e.g., running from a house fire) these mechanisms may save your life. When you're simply battling traffic they could increase your risk of heart attack, ulcers, diabetes, even death, depending on how often you're facing the stress.

Once the crisis has passed, your body moves into the second, or *recuperative,* stage, when damage sustained during alarm is repaired. Your body heads back to normal levels of heart rate and blood pressure. Systems begin to normalize. Depending on the severity of the stress, recuperation may take minutes or hours.

The final stage, when the body returns to its normal state, is called *relaxed alertness,* or the relaxation response.

Your goal after every stressful situation should be to give your body enough time to recover through proper nutrition, rest and relaxation. That's not always how it works, is it?

Acute stressful events compete with a whole host of psychological and technological stressors that happen with such frequency that we don't have time to recuperate between them. The result is chronic stress – a continual stress state with little or no recuperation.

**Acute Stress:** *Single bouts of stressful events with adequate recuperation in between.*

**Chronic Stress:** *Stress without recuperation.*

Unfortunately, increased life pressures make it more difficult to avoid stress so many of us live in a perpetual state of frazzle.

At 6:00 a.m. your alarm clock blares and shocks you out of sleep. Your heart is racing right out of the gate and despite your fatigue you crawl out of bed and get on with your day.

Get the kids ready for school, make breakfast, make lunches, get yourself ready for work. You drop the kids off at school then fight traffic all the way to your office. Almost late.

You fight to find parking, you stress about how much it costs, your cell phone has already started ringing, and by the time you get to your office you have forty emails that need your attention.

Phone ringing, meetings to attend, co-workers who need your help, projects that must get done today, go, go, go, go.

Skip lunch, miss your workout, fuel up on coffee and muffins, phone still ringing until the end of the day.

Back in traffic, pick up the kids, drop them off at their activities, pick up groceries, check in with your aging mother, pick up the kids and get home to make dinner. Go, go, go, go.

Dinner, clean up, laundry, kids' homework, one last check on email, call your sister, time with your spouse, time with your dog, time for yourself. Go, go, go, gone.

## CHRONIC STRESS, ENERGY AND CREATIVITY

The stressors that hit you in a day may show up as one hundred seemingly minor stressors, but without time to recover your body will eventually feel the stress in a bigger way.

In a chronic stress environment your body wages a tug-of-war between the stress response and relaxation response, trying desperately to find peace. The stress hormone cortisol is in the middle of that battle.

In a chronic stress state the physiological stress that enters your body doesn't leave you. Your body must then contend with higher than normal levels of cortisol over longer periods of time.

High blood pressure, high blood sugar, high gastric secretions, and a confused immune function will eventually conspire to make you sick, tired and uninspired.

Prolonged presence of cortisol can also decrease bone density and muscle tissue over time, and increase abdominal fat, which is associated with health problems like heart attack, stroke and high levels of bad cholesterol.

Perhaps the most interesting side effect of chronic stress and ever present cortisol is its impact on creativity.

In a stress state our cognitive function becomes impaired. Remember that the stress response prepares the body for fight or flight, and in survival mode the brain doesn't care about being creative or innovative, it just wants to get through the stress.

If you're regularly stressed your energy and productivity will take a nose dive. In times like this it's relaxation and recuperation that will have you energized and firing on all creative cylinders once again.

## STRESS AWARENESS

Despite its ever-presence, it seems stress is quite difficult to define. What is stressful to you may be enjoyable or even energizing for someone else. How you react — emotionally, behaviorally and physically — to stressful situations may be quite different than how a friend, co-worker or spouse reacts.

The first defense against stress is to acknowledge its presence and increase your awareness about how it manifests in your life. Determine what really causes you stress. How does your body respond?

Financial challenges, work deadlines, a challenging co-worker, struggles with your rebellious teen, poor health — whatever they are, identify them and pay attention to how you respond to stress when it's present.

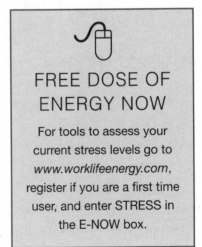

**FREE DOSE OF ENERGY NOW**

For tools to assess your current stress levels go to *www.worklifeenergy.com*, register if you are a first time user, and enter STRESS in the E-NOW box.

Stress shows up as emotional, behavioral and physical signs in response to events around us. Emotional signs of stress include:

- Mood swings
- Lack of enthusiasm
- Feeling angry or guilty
- Feeling nervous, apprehensive, anxious
- Feelings of helplessness and lack of control
- Loss of confidence
- Lack of self-esteem
- Inability to concentrate

You've likely experienced one or all of the signs during times of stress. When the workload becomes overwhelming or a problem seems too big to handle it is normal to feel nervous or helpless. It makes sense that enthusiasm might falter in the face of a stressful experience. It's not at all uncommon for confidence and self-esteem to take a beating either.

When these emotional signs make their presence known, we're often in the middle of the stress that created them so instead of addressing them we ignore them – and yes, that adds to your stress. If you haven't noticed them already, you'll soon see behavioral signs creeping in which include:

- Accident proneness
- Increased smoking, drug, or alcohol use
- Overeating or loss of appetite
- Poor quality sleep
- Withdrawal from supportive relationships
- Being too busy to relax
- Poor time management
- Impaired performance at work or home
- Not looking after yourself

It shouldn't come as a surprise. Inability to deal with the difficult emotional feelings associated with stress often leads to stuffing them into distracting, often destructive behaviors.

As stress increases you might start smoking or reach for comfort foods. You might drink more to calm your nerves, sleep too much or not enough, work more, forgo relaxation, and ignore simple self-care practices.

Unfortunately this pattern of pushing past the signs will inevitably lead to physical distress in the body, and you want to avoid this at all costs.

Physical signs of stress include:

- Headaches
- Extreme fatigue
- Stomach or back pains
- Digestive distress
- Jaw or neck pain
- Weight gain
- High blood pressure
- Chest pains

All of the above physical signs of stress will not only bring you discomfort and pain, but they are all precursors to more serious and life-threatening health concerns if left unchecked. It's important to recognize their arrival and do what you can to minimize their impact, not only to avoid illness, but to simply feel better and more energetic.

## STRESS DEFENSE

While we usually have a good idea about what causes our stress, we don't often take the time to really dissect our stress, and it can be a helpful process. To defend yourself against rising stress, consider the following.

### Recognize what you can change.

*When faced with a stressful situation can you minimize the impact by walking away or avoiding the stress?* I'm not suggesting you run away from your problems, but in some situations where the stress is ongoing and unavoidable – a difficult co-worker, a high-traffic route to the office, or an unnecessary meeting, for example — stress can be minimized by avoiding a person or place or choosing a different option.

*Can you reduce the intensity of the things that cause you stress?* Instead of trying to slay the beast in one day is it possible to manage it over several days or even weeks? Chip away at a dreaded task rather than procrastinating until it becomes insurmountable. If it is unmanageable, can you ask for help?

*Can you shorten your exposure to stress?* If you know you have a particularly stressful work day or event, can you build in breaks or even leave the premises for short intervals through the day? Can you schedule meetings with challenging clients all on one day so the stress isn't spread over several days?

And perhaps the most important question to ask yourself is: *Can I devote the time and energy it will take to de-stress my life?* Can you? If stress is something that has a grip on your life, how badly do you want that to end?

Set some goals regarding what you'd like to change, take small steps toward the goals, structure your time so you're not overscheduled, and ask for help.

## Mind your emotional reactions to stress.

The stress response is triggered by your perception of a particular situation and your ability to cope with it. You may or may not be accurate in your appraisal.

*When faced with a potential stressor, do you make mountains out of molehills?* There's a clever quote by Mark Twain that speaks to this. *I've lived through some terrible things in my life, some of which actually happened.* We create unnecessary stress for ourselves by anticipating stress that may or may not occur. Prepare yourself with options but focus on positive outcomes.

*Do you overreact and view things as absolutely critical and urgent?* If so, attempt to adopt more moderate views; try to see the stress as something you can cope with rather than something that overpowers you.

*Are you expecting to please everyone?* This can be a great source of stress, partly because it robs you of time that could be focused on your goals, but mostly because it's near impossible to figure out what everyone around you might actually need. It's an exercise in insanity. First, look out for #1.

## Know your physical reactions to stress.

We've already established that some level of stress will always be present in your life. When it is, don't let it run you down.

Stress has the capacity to elevate certain physiological functions, like heart rate and blood pressure. Many people are hot reactors to stressful events and will react to a boiling point when stress hits.

When the going gets *really* tough try slow, deep breathing to bring heart rate and respiration back to normal. Count to ten as you do.

Try relaxation techniques to reduce muscle tension. First tighten the muscles in your neck and shoulders, clench your fists, tighten your abdominals and hold your breath. Second, release all the tension as you exhale your breath.

Listen to relaxation techniques on audio. Meditation and other mind body practices, like yoga, can also help *calm the rushing mind.*

## Build your resilience against stress.

Because stress impacts the physical body in so many big and small ways, one of the best things you can do to combat stress is to maintain your health and vitality. Period. It's what this book is all about really – small steps to an energetic life – and since physical health staves off so many energy-sucking entities, including stress, let me remind you once again.

*Eat well-balanced, nutritious meals.* Stress thrives on sugar and caffeine. Instead, choose healthy, balanced meals with regular snacks throughout the day. Keep your blood sugars level to increase your energy, promote clear thinking, and enhance your coping mechanisms.

*Avoid nicotine, excessive caffeine, and other stimulants.* First of all, do I really have to remind you not to smoke? Yes, nicotine in the blood stream may make you feel calm in the moment. It also acts as a stimulant to the brain. Talk about mixed signals.

Well, if that's not enough, may I remind you that cigarette smoke contains over 4,000 chemicals, including 43 known cancer-causing compounds and 400 other toxins. These include nicotine, tar, and carbon monoxide, as well as formaldehyde, ammonia, hydrogen cyanide, arsenic, and DDT – none of which are part of living a healthy, energetic life. You can tell me to butt out if I'm nagging you, but I'd rather you did.

Caffeine may not be so unhealthy, but since it's a stimulant it will add to your stress state and make your feel more agitated when you need to seek calm. Stimulants like energy drinks or even pills to help you stay alert will do the same and place unnecessary stress on your heart.

*Get enough sleep.* Sleep deprivation is a form of stress. Your body will react to excess fatigue in much the same way it will react to the stress of being late for a meeting or writing a difficult exam. Not only will your fatigue and mounting stress add wear and tear to your body, but it will seriously affect your ability to cope in the moment. If you're serious about stress reduction get serious about sleep.

*Laugh more.* There aren't many things that can make you feel as good as a hearty belly laugh, and there are so many wonderful health benefits that take place in your body when you laugh.

A really good laugh increases your heart rate and oxygen supply, stimulates blood circulation, and helps ease muscle tension.

Laughter decreases stress hormones and increases immune cells and infection-fighting antibodies, all of which will improve your resistance to disease.

Laughter triggers the release of positive endorphins that flood your body with natural feel-good chemicals that boost your wellbeing and can even temporarily relieve pain.

> If you feel your coping mechanisms breaking down, stop in the moment and check in with the acronym H.A.L.T.:
>
> **H**ungry
> **A**ngry
> **L**onely
> **T**ired
>
> Sometimes our ability to cope may be affected by a simple need for fuel, an unresolved grievance that is stealing our focus, a need for social connection after too much isolation, or a plain old nap. It some cases it's unnecessary to overthink your stress. HALT and do what it takes to feel better.

Beyond the physical benefits there are a number of mental benefits to laughter as well. It's difficult to feel anxious, irritated, or upset when you're laughing. Laughter reduces stress and increases energy, helping you stay focused and productive. And, of course, when you allow humor into a situation it allows you to see things in a more realistic, less threatening light. Lighten up baby!

*Get regular exercise.* It's like a broken record, isn't it? Is there anything that physical activity doesn't improve?

Regular exercise has been known to reduce the severity of the stress response, shorten the recovery time from stress, and reduce stress-related vulnerability to disease. If life is so busy that you're not able to fit in adequate recuperation between stressful events, exercise can help!

When you complain that you are too busy or stressed to exercise, remind yourself that beyond the health benefits, even one bout of activity can work to provide distraction from the day's challenges. A visit to the gym can help you feel good and regain some of the control the work day may have robbed from you.

It's important to note however that exercise itself is a stressor, so when stress is really high, exercise should lean toward moderate or mild levels of activity. A walk outdoors or a meditative swim will bring more calming benefits in these instances than a high-intensity cardio kickboxing class or a killer attack on the treadmill.

## Maintain your emotional reserves.

When stress gets out of hand, gain support from those around you. When you're overwhelmed the tendency can be to retreat and hide, or gloss over the seriousness of your stress. Why go it alone?

*Develop your support network.* I think we all need what I call a *2a.m. friend*: that person you know so well you can call them at any time of the day, even 2 in the morning. Friends give you perspective and support. And when you talk through your stress, its impact is often lessened.

Pursue realistic, fulfilling goals. Goals can energize you if they're in line with your desires and values, and can create stress if they're not. For stress-free goal setting, make sure the dreams and plans you're going after are in fact yours and not someone else's. Set big goals for sure, and be realistic in your pursuit of them.

You're on your way to great improvements with stress management. You've made a commitment to exercise more, take small bites with healthy eating, and even improve your sleep habits. Changes like these will be rewarding in time but can be stressful too.

Recognize that change takes time. In the face of setbacks, stay strong. Realign your compass and get back on track without beating yourself up.

Every small step you take toward better physical health will go a long way to reducing your stress and improving the quality of your life, mind, body and spirit.

## CHARGE!

Part 2 of this book is all about living a more energetic life by taking care of your body. The last piece of that puzzle is to minimize your stress.

First accept that stress is an unwelcome part of your life, and then allow yourself the time and focus to do something about it.

What causes you stress? Get a blank piece of paper and write it all down. Be specific. It's not enough to write *My job causes me stress.* You'll gain more problem solving traction by honing in on the exact aspects of your job that add to your stress: *My workload at month's end is enough for two people to do.*

Don't stress about creating a tidy list of stressors, just brainstorm and get it all out on paper.

Now look at the list. Do your stressors pile up at work, home or both? Are they related to people or circumstances? If you had to pick one or two items on the list that blow the roof off your stress, which would win and what can you do about them?

Stress won't go away over night, but if you identify the sources of your stress you can devise a plan to minimize or eliminate at least some of your stress.

Take action on your stress – even in small steps – and watch your energy soar!

## WHATEVER IT TAKES

Confessions of a stress case: *Some days it just feels like the stress is inescapable. There is just too much to do and not enough time to do it – forget doing it well. Most of the time I find myself white knuckling through the day, just waiting for it to end, and I certainly don't look forward to getting up the next day. I snap at my kids, I ignore my spouse, and I can't remember the last time I felt calm. I hate being this stressed but I don't have the time or energy to do anything about it!*

When it comes to managing stress, the biggest challenge I hear from audience members and clients is the lack of time and energy to slay the stress beast. Despite this truth, the negative impact of stress on mind, body and spirit should not be ignored.

If stress is high and time and energy are low, don't wait until that changes; it won't. You may not be able to control the stress coming in, but you do have 100 percent control over strengthening your physical body against it.

Take small steps to boost your resilience, starting now. Try the following daily resilience boosters for one week and see how you feel:

1. Eat a healthy breakfast, preferably not on the go.

2. Reduce or eliminate caffeine consumption, especially after midday.

3. Drink lots of water. Skip soda entirely.

4. Walk outside for ten minutes every day. I know you're busy, but it's only ten minutes.

5. Leave work on time at least two days this week.

6. When you feel your blood pressure rising take a few deep, slow breaths of air.

7. Snack healthfully throughout the day.

8. Minimize alcohol consumption. It's only for one week. Give it a go.

9. Go to bed one hour earlier at least two nights this week.

10. Hug your loved ones every day, morning and night.

Each of the suggestions above really shouldn't be that difficult to implement if you're serious about knocking down your stress. Ahhh, resilience. It's as easy as counting to ten. *Do whatever it takes.*

## ENERGY NOW!

### Stress Stoppers

- Diffuse misunderstandings before they happen by talking things over with the person in question.
- Walk away from the stressful situation and cool down before reacting.
- Use regular exercise as one method of stress management. It's a good one!
- Don't be afraid to say *I'm sorry* if you make a mistake.
- Schedule down-time into your calendar. A few twenty-to-thirty-minute open slots per day provide flexibility against surprises.
- Set your watch five to ten minutes ahead to avoid the stress of being late.
- Rubbed the wrong way? Count to ten before you speak.
- Take time to recover, refocus and regenerate after a major event like a divorce, relocation, promotion, or birth of a child.
- Break down big problems into smaller parts (e.g., answer one letter or phone call per day), instead of dealing with everything at once.
- Talk through your troubles. It can help you blow off steam and gain the perspective you need to solve the problem more easily.
- Sit back and sip some chamomile tea. It promotes relaxation and reduces anxiety.
- Drive in the slow lane or avoid busy roads to help you stay calm while driving.

- Be realistic about your expectations of yourself at work and in life. Pursuit of perfection only causes stress.
- Smell the flowers, hug someone you love, or smile at your neighbor.
- Breathe. Count to four as you inhale, and again as you exhale.
- Own your power. Remind yourself that you are in control of the events in your life. Choose a happy ending.

# PART 3

## Feed Your Spirit

PHYSICAL HEALTH IS A CRUCIAL PART OF THE *Energy Now!* equation and it will certainly provide you with resilience to cope with all that life throws your way. If you've read the last five chapters you're armed with many ways to energize your body.

By taking small steps to improve your fitness, nutrition, hydration, sleep and stress, you'll be well on your way to a healthy and energetic life. Nice work.

Now it's time to shift gears and tap into a whole other wicked and wonderful energy source within you. It's what I call spiritual energy and I believe it holds an unlimited supply of life-affirming, fun-generating energy if you connect to it well.

In this case I prefer to define spirituality as *tapping into your spirit's reality* – looking deep within head and heart to the things that sustain your spirit.

If exercise, good nutrition, sleep, and stress management improve your physical energy, then spiritual energy is impacted by the ways you take care of yourself socially, emotionally, and spiritually – through interacting meaningfully with other people, doing things you love, being inspired and creative, building self-confidence, being hopeful, giving and receiving love and valuing yourself.

I'll admit it's a deep rabbit hole to jump into but I think head and heart are worth exploring for the abundance of energy and vitality hidden there.

The next three chapters will touch on different aspects of emotional energy in a section I've labelled *Feed your Spirit* – so open your wings and take flight.

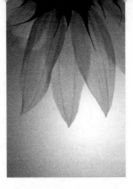

CHAPTER 10

# The Happiness Factor

*Each morning when I open my eyes I say to myself:*
*I, not events, have the power to make me happy or*
*unhappy today. I can choose which it shall be.*
*Yesterday is dead, tomorrow hasn't arrived yet. I have*
*just one day, today, and I'm going to be happy in it.*
—GROUCHO MARX

A H, happiness – an enduring life goal. Though money can't buy it, it's at the root of success and fulfillment. Happy people are more likely to work toward goals, seek out the resources they need, and draw people in with their liveliness and optimism – key building blocks of success. And happy people always seem to have more energy. That thought makes me happy.

Happiness is one of our more treasured emotions for what it represents and how it makes us feel, and yet it can be so hard to embrace fully. The simple pursuit of happiness gets rerouted by day-to-day busyness, expectations from others, demands you place on yourself, and of course enduring fatigue.

Happiness has to engage in the daily tug-of-war against sadness, indifference and doubt. It gets mixed up in a swirling pot of emotional energy that we have to sort and prioritize before we get it right, before we truly embrace or even understand true happiness.

Emotional energy has the power to pull you in two extreme directions: down with feelings of hopelessness or depression, or *up* with feelings of hope, empowerment and happiness.

You know the negative side of this equation if you've allowed someone to walk all over you, or you've stopped prioritizing your own hobbies. You also know the up-side if you've ever felt the bliss of real love, or accomplished a treasured goal.

In her book *The Emotional Energy Factor*, Mira Kirshenbaum states that as much as 70 percent of our total energy is emotional – the kind that manifests from the things I mention above. If that's the case, then even the most rigid physical health plan won't guarantee an energetic life. We need to also look within.

Emotional energy encompasses all of the positive and negative feelings we carry with us every day – emotions like happiness, sadness, anger, guilt, fear, surprise, interest, and enthusiasm.

Sadly, when life gets stressful and busy, it's easier to get pulled toward negative emotions – especially if physical energy is already low, and even when it's not. You can do all the right things with your physical health and still be sucked dry of energy if your emotional health is poor. Since a big part of positive emotional energy is connected to your personal happiness, let's start there.

## THE LEAKY TOILET TEST

Throughout the year, in an effort to conserve water, my city broadcasts public service messages asking residents to take the *leaky toilet test*. You may not know it's happening, but older toilets can silently leak gallons of water because of loose valves and worn stoppers.

They tell us to put a few drops of food coloring into the toilet bowl and wait. If the initial bright color eventually fades it means the toilet is leaking water unnecessarily.

Your happiness can drain from you in a similar subtle fashion. As you rush busily through your day you may not always be aware of the emotional energy drains that are slowly emptying your tank or you may ignore them rather than face the pain. Either way, if you hope to regain those feelings of happiness and hope then it's time to source out the leaks.

If some aspect of your life – big or small – is out of whack, you can't ignore it and expect it to go away. It will eventually overshadow even the good things that are happening in your life. This is not to say that you can't be happy and challenged at the same time, but your true potential will be slowed until the leak gets filled.

If your finances are stretched and you're not doing anything about it; if you're in an unhappy or unfulfilled relationship; if you're not satisfied with your work; if you're dissatisfied with your health; if you're in conflict with any person, thought process or circumstance, that conflict will get in the way of realizing ultimate happiness and success.

And you know the difference, don't you? It's about honouring who you are and what you believe in. It's at the root of happiness.

## Happiness and Your Values

Emotional energy and happiness are at their highest when you identify and honor your values. Values are those things that really matter to you – the ideas and beliefs you hold special.

Values like respect, authenticity, trust, integrity and caring, when exploited – by you or others – manifest over time into feelings of stress, disappointment, disbelief, low self-esteem, poor self-worth, and unhappiness.

I can't believe I let him say that to me.
Why wasn't I more careful with my money?
I am so mad at myself for letting my health go.
What a fool I am. I thought I could trust her.
I'm capable of so much more than this.
Why can't I learn to say no?
Why don't I work harder?
I thought he loved me.
I knew she'd let me down.

## FREE DOSE OF ENERGY NOW

What values are important to you? Go to *www.worklifeenergy.com*. Register if you are a first time user, enter VALUES in the E-NOW box, and access an exercise to help you get clear on your values.

I'm so stupid for not seeing it in the first place.

Every time your values are tested another crack shows up in your energy tank and a little more of your happiness and self-worth drips away. You're worth so much more than that.

## POSITIVE IDENTIFICATION

Your happiness is impacted by external experiences and interactions as well as your own internal thoughts and perceptions. And what a battle they can wage. Let's identify sources of a few of our biggest leaks.

Rather than dwell on the energy leak that you're attempting to move away from, I've spun the list to identify the positive behavior to strive for.

### Set Meaningful Goals

I talked about writing a book for nearly ten years. It frustrated me because I knew I could do it...so why didn't I? Last year two of my speaker colleagues invited me into their book writing workshop and I figured it was my only chance.

Susan, an accomplished author, would help us set goals and mentor us, and we would all hold each other accountable. Once this process began, the book I talked about for ten years – this book – came to life in just over a year. It's been hard work, but *what a feeling!*

Happiness and fulfillment are fed by accomplishment. It's important to always have something in your plans to strive toward. It gives you a reason to get out of bed every day. If you've been cruising along without trying something new, give your values a shake.

Sign up for a running race, plan that trip to Europe, start that blog you've been talking about, take that class, write that book. It's energizing to have something to look forward to.

## Take Responsibility for Your Life

In Chapter 3 I state quite bluntly: *If your life sucks, it's your fault.* If you need to be reminded of my candor, flip back to page 62.

You are the common denominator in every aspect of your life that isn't working. You can ignore that and continue to let your emotional energy drain away, or you can face up to it and admit that the fix is nobody's responsibility but yours.

No more excuses. No more blaming the boss, the kids, the circumstances, lack of finances, time, or motivation. Take responsibility for your life.

If you need to get a job or be better with money, do it. If you have health issues that cause you and those around you unnecessary stress, do everything in your power to get help. Look at the leaks and get serious about getting them filled. You're the only one who can get that job done, so do it.

You know you're capable of big things. Pay close attention to the situations in your life where you may be holding yourself back. Look at your life from a different vantage point.

And remember, you are also the common denominator in every aspect of your life that is fun, fabulous and fulfilling and I bet there's more there than you know. Jump in and get that energy flowing again.

## Do a Toxic People Dump

Why do you keep spending time with people who bring you down? What do you gain from listening endlessly to that co-worker's complaints and negativity? How would your life change if you stopped pandering to that friend's endless needy requests? And why would you spend another minute with that ambitionless low-life just because you're afraid of being alone?

Let's face it, some people in our lives can only be described as toxic. Their mission in life is to feel better about their lives by poisoning yours. They do that by treating you poorly, taking advantage of your good nature, or sucking away your energy with their neediness. Who died and made you martyr? You deserve better.

Instead, surround yourself with competent, responsible and supportive people who believe in you and want good things for you. People like this will make you feel good about yourself and inspire you to do and be more, and they won't even expect anything in return. Well, except for the chance to see you truly happy.

## Let Go of the Past

To truly live in the moment is something that is very hard for many of us. We hang too much energy on a lost friendship. We stew for months over a co-worker's indiscretion. We dwell on the hardships of a painful divorce, or mourn far too long for a deceased loved one.

Yes, it can be hard to let go, but these types of attachments deplete your emotional energy and get in the way of today.

The best revenge for a painful separation is to live a fabulous life. The "friend" you lost was likely worth losing. Go find a better one. And if you have no control over an individual or a situation, quit driving yourself crazy over it. Remind yourself why these circumstances were so difficult and try to move on.

In matters of grief, allow yourself time to mourn. It's healthy. Cry all your tears for your deceased loved one and then ask yourself, *What would they wish for me?* Live that life. They're watching over you, so make them proud.

## Please Yourself

Just because someone asks you to do it, doesn't mean you have to say yes. Your mother may believe she knows best, but you're an adult now and you can do as you please. And so what if there's no one else to do it; it's not in *your* job description. No one appointed *you* martyr to the masses. And while we're at it, quit worrying about what everyone will think of your decisions. They're your decisions.

Do what you want to do. Be the person you know you are deep down inside. Quit giving your energy away to keep everybody else happy. Keep it for yourself. You're an amazing person. But you knew that already.

## Green your Own Grass

Oh, it's tough to look at the Joneses and realize you just can't keep up. Your co-worker only has to look at a treadmill to lose weight. Your neighbor always seems to be jetting off on great vacations and you're sure he makes less than you. Your friends find love so easily and you stay single. A bigger house, a better promotion, a great relationship, a sparkling smile – the grass is always greener *over there*.

You want what they want and you can't help but feel a tinge of envy, but is your life really that bad? Focus your energy on the successes and accomplishments of others and that's exactly where it will end up.

Why not come back to your side of the fence and *green your own grass*. Redirect your energy toward the good things in your life. Work toward your goals without comparing yourself to every Tom, Dick and Mary around you. The pressure is off. Enjoy the ride.

## Don't Worry

If you're a chronic worrier, this is easier said than done, but when you dwell excessively on what *might* happen or worry about things that are out of your control, energy drains with every catastrophic thought.

Many 12-step programs embrace *The Serenity Prayer* as a guide in these circumstances. It's a powerful appeal worth remembering:

> *God, grant me the serenity to accept the things*
> *I cannot change, the courage to change the things*
> *I can and the wisdom to know the difference.*

If you're losing sleep over something out of your control, let it go. It's all you can do.

If your worry is about something that you do have the means to change, then take action. Your problem may not be solved quickly, but if you take one small step in the direction of change you'll replace worry with empowerment and gain energy to take another step.

## Say You're Sorry

Guilt is a powerful emotion that will hang around your neck like the albatross from Samuel Taylor Coleridge's *The Rime of the Ancient*

*Mariner,* slowly weighing you down and infecting those around you with its stench. If that's not energy sucking, I don't know what is.

If you're feeling guilt or remorse over something you said or did, make amends — even if it's with yourself. There is nothing more powerful than a genuine apology or heartfelt explanation. Try it if you don't believe me. Let go of guilt and feel the surge of energy that follows.

## Take Care of You

I won't belabor this point because it's what this book is all about, but when you stop taking care of yourself the flow of energy in your life shuts down quickly and for so many reasons.

Your personal health is your number one responsibility, even above childcare and family responsibilities. Don't fight me on this. It is.

When you stop taking care of yourself you gain weight, your health weakens, you have less energy and you certainly don't feel very good about yourself. This is not the kind of example you want to be for your loved ones.

Get regular exercise, take time for yourself, set a good example for your family. Love yourself more and you'll have more energy and love to pass on to those close to you.

## Do What Makes You Happy

Happiness has an interesting energy, doesn't it? We connect it to other people — what they say or do or believe, and how they treat us. We connect it to material possessions, often with the mistaken belief that this will bring us happiness. We attach it to our accomplishments, money, and experiences in an endless search for a little more.

It's true that all of these things can add to your happiness, but none will bring you as much as the kind that is connected to what you value and believe in. I hope you're feeling it. If you're not there yet, read on and take the steps to find true happiness for yourself.

## CHARGE!

What makes you happy? What are the things in your life, significant or silly, that bring you joy? A few of the things on my list include sunny days, reaching a goal, snowboarding, digging in my garden, walking by the river with my sweetie and my dog, or cooking a great meal together. If I'm doing any of those things, I usually feel pretty content.

Write your HAPPINESS list. Do it now.

Do something from this list every day. Brilliant!

## WHATEVER IT TAKES (*Unhappy Me*)

Several years ago one of my personal training clients fired me. She told me she had benefited from my workouts, but lately the energy I was bringing to our sessions was bringing her down. She could tell I was unhappy and unfulfilled with some aspect of my life, and even though I thought I was covering it up, she felt it and it was sucking her dry.

She wanted the best for me though, so she hugged me as a concerned parent might, and gave me the name of her counsellor. *Get some help* she told me. *You'll feel better.* It was hard to hear, but she was right. I was unhappy and I had been for a while. If I couldn't figure it out on my own, what was the harm in asking for help?

If you've ever struggled through an unhappy period in your life or experienced depression on any level, you know that it drains you of energy very quickly. No matter how fit and healthy you may be at the time, unhappiness will rob you of vitality and get-up-and-go more quickly than exercise and healthy eating can bring it back.

I started to see a counsellor once a week. Talk about opening up a Pandora's box of hurts that needed healing. It was difficult at first – this *finding myself* – but anything worth having is worth working for.

Being bullied in high school, walking away from Olympic possibilities, dealing with my dad's death, realizing how that affected my relationships, struggling with career decisions, understanding my self-worth issues, coming to terms with life as it was – why would I think myself immune to these life events?

When I was in the middle of dealing with my issues, my counsellor would often remind me *you're not always going to feel this way.* I didn't believe her at first but I persevered, and eventually the clouds opened up and I started to see the light. It was brimming in hope and happiness by the way.

If you're unhappy, can you ask for help? If you can't afford to see a professional, is there a trusted friend or family member you can talk with? You don't deserve to feel this way any longer. Happiness is a wellspring of energy that will bring so much more to life once you harness its true power. Do whatever it takes.

## ENERGY NOW!

### The Happiness Factor

- Make a list of everything that makes you happy, no matter how small.
- Smile at yourself in the mirror every morning.
- Call a friend who makes you laugh.
- Make a date with yourself at least every month. Do something you love.
- Watch your favorite comedy or feel-good movie.
- End a conflict with someone you love.
- Talk through your troubles with a trusted confidante.
- Do something off your happiness list.
- Spend some time in nature.
- Ask for help if you're struggling with something.
- Write a gratitude list before you go to sleep.
- Read it again when you wake up.
- Emulate your beloved pet's unconditional love.

- Challenge yourself in one small way today.
- Do something that gets your heart racing in a good way.
- Listen to uplifting music. Dance if the urge hits you.
- Ask your best friend to tell you what they like about you. Soak it in.
- Why wait for someone else to think of it? Buy yourself flowers.
- What (or who) makes you laugh? You can never get enough good giggles.
- Your favorite person wants some of your time today. Give it to them.
- My dog Lilly has my heart. Pets are an endless source of happiness. Get one, borrow one, love one.
- When was the last time you laughed until your belly hurt? Ooo, that's energizing!
- Having a tough day? Smile and fool your face. Eventually your mindset will catch up.
- Life's too short. Lighten up. Buy a clown nose and wear it to work.
- What if you stopped with all of the negative thinking and focused on fun? That's FUN!
- If you spend even a small part of each day in the pursuit of happy, life will be good. That's a happy thought.

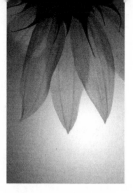

CHAPTER 11

# The Kindness Experiment

*I've learned that people will forget what you said,
people will forget what you did, but people will
never forget how you made them feel.*
—Maya Angelou

MAKE love, not war. Give peace a chance. Love thy neighbor. Can't we all just get along?

Imagine a world where everyone is just a *little* kinder. The people you pass on the street look you in the eye and say *good morning*. You take the time to help your elderly neighbor unpack their groceries. As you step up to buy your morning coffee you find out the person ahead of you secretly paid for it. When shopping, you allow a person in a hurry to go ahead of you in the checkout line. As you merge into traffic the driver ahead lets you in. You do the same for someone else and they wave *thank you*. You get to your office and your co-worker compliments you on the great job you're doing. You get home and your partner tells you how much they appreciate you.

What a wonderful world it would be if we all got along just a little better.

Social wellness or connectedness to other people is such an important part of a happy, healthy life, and it's also a major part of the big energy picture. Kindness is energizing.

*Kindness as an energy source?* You better believe it! Social wellness comes from developing healthy relationships with family, friends, co-workers and society as a whole, and that's not always an easy thing to do.

I'll admit that when life gets busy it's far easier to rush through the day with my head down, avoiding eye-contact and potential interruptions along the way – especially with people I don't really know.

It's quicker and more efficient to just get to the point and get on with it. People and interactions slow you down, after all. It may be true but it doesn't seem like much fun.

If you want to live a more energetic life you should try to get along with everyone. Make efforts to connect authentically with people throughout your day – with loved ones, friends, co-workers and even strangers. Yes, I realize this may seem like a big effort to make when energy is low, but there's a good reason for it.

## PEOPLE POWER

There is an energy exchange that happens between people that can be good, bad, or somewhere in between. Every human being you come in contact with every day has the capacity to impact your personal energy in a positive direction or a negative one. You have the same influence with the people you interact with every day.

We exchange energy through words, body language, eye contact, tone of voice and mere presence. Energy is exchanged positively through a loving glance or tender touch, through kind words and gestures, a smile or a laugh, or a helpful act. Think about the people in your life with whom you interact in these ways and how wonderful that makes you feel.

Energy is exchanged negatively through a grimace or frown, a threatening word or unfriendly gesture, through aggression, a hurtful act or mere indifference. You've likely experienced this type of interaction with people around you as well. It doesn't feel as good, does it? How do you connect with other people and what kind of energy do you spread? When you choose kindness over judgment or indifference, everybody wins.

## Kindness, Acceptance or Tolerance

*Yeah, but I really don't like that person.* Okay, so maybe it's a bit much to expect you to be kind to everyone around you all the time. There are people in our lives that for whatever reason just rub us the wrong way. I call them *fork* people.

> *If you don't like someone, the way they hold their fork will make you furious; if you do like them, they can turn their plate over in your lap and you won't mind.*
> —IRVING BECKER

Even as adults we accept and reject people from our circle of friends based on sometimes arbitrary facts, and that can create real tension.

So, what to do? If you don't like someone, the first option is to get to know them better. That's not an easy thing to do if you already hold a negative judgment against them, but sometimes it can be an eye-opening experience.

## Seek First to Understand

I once worked with a woman who drove me crazy with her controlling and negative behavior. I was new on the job and had been hired to offset her growing workload, so you'd think she'd be happy to have me on board. She wasn't.

I was right out of university and was keen to do a good job. I was full of ideas and energy that she simply did not appreciate, and she let me know as often as she could. *It's not how we do things around here. I've been in this position for fifteen years so how about you listen to me? I'm not about to implement a bunch of ideas that I know won't work anyway.* When I spoke up in meetings she would roll her eyes or grunt from her spot at the table. If I did something well she'd chalk it up to luck and was unable to extend a compliment. She didn't like me, so I did what any open-minded-kindness-loving individual might do. I didn't like her back.

We entered into a push and pull tug-of-war of a working relationship that made it painful to go to work. We argued all the time, tossed sarcasm out at every turn, and had nothing nice to say about the other when we gossiped to co-workers.

We didn't support each other; in fact, we made every effort to thwart success for the other – so much so that our boss brought in a mediator to help us get along. True story.

If you don't like someone, get to know them better. I was forced into it but I did get to know her better. Through our counseling sessions I eventually came to understand her resistance toward me and learned a few things about myself too.

She had worked solo in this job for over fifteen years and all of a sudden a fresh-faced university kid comes into the picture, tossing inexperience and over-exuberance in her face.

On the one hand she felt threatened because I had new ideas, fresh energy and a university education, and on the other hand she felt disrespected because she knew a lot and had much to teach me if I'd only let her.

It was all true. She had been shut down to my ideas. I had been shut down to learning from her. We both needed to drop our guards and accept each other as we were. When we did, everything changed.

She was actually a really nice person. She actually knew a lot more than I gave her credit for. I could actually learn from her. She was funny, hard-working and very good at her job. It's amazing the things that you can see when your eyes aren't clouded by judgment. I had been arrogant and closed-minded.

The best part was that when we put our heads together and worked as a team, we had a great time and achieved great things. We became friends.

## Lessons from the Playground

*I could spend a lifetime getting to know this person and nothing would change.* Admittedly we all have at least one *fork person* in our lives that no amount of patience and understanding will impact. Fair enough. In these instances I ask you to think back to something you likely learned in kindergarten. If you have nothing nice to say, don't say anything at all.

Don't engage. Don't provoke. Just zip it.

This concept often meets with push back when I mention it in my presentations as people try to convince me of the merit of putting someone in their place. Why? So you can hang out in all that negative energy for just a little bit longer?

When you judge other people, it's like drinking poison and expecting the other person to die.

As you toss out each bad thought or discrimination toward the object of your disdain there is a 100-percent chance you'll get to experience the negative feelings associated with that exchange.

Your recipient may or may not decide that what you have to say is worthy of owning. Your judgments may fall on deaf ears or you may get an earful back. Either way, you're assured of hanging in the negative space for a good long while. Just so you can be right. That is not my idea of fun.

## Would You Rather Be Right or Happy?

Sometimes it's best to choose the moral high ground over conflict. This is not about being the model of goodness and righteousness; it's to preserve the sphere of social wellness around you. Choose kindness. It just feels better.

In doing so you'll begin to attract other positive people into your realm. Conflict is exhausting. Harmony is energizing.

When kindness seems impossible, try to embrace acceptance or tolerance as your default. Your silent smile is one small affirming interaction you give to the world.

## Home Is Where the Heart Is

It's sad to say, but sometimes we show the greatest impatience and intolerance to the people closest to us.

You may snap at your teenager and call him lazy. You might speak to your spouse with a sarcastic tone. You could raise your voice impatiently at your messy toddler. Would you communicate with a coworker or total stranger this way? I don't think so.

So often we give our best energy to our jobs, co-workers, and people we interact with during the day. The people we love the most get us at our worst – at the end of the day with an empty energy tank and low patience threshold. The circumstances should be reversed.

If you find yourself snapping at your sweetie or getting cranky with your kids, maybe it's time for a kindness intervention.

Lack of energy is a key perpetrator, but so is lack of awareness. Pay attention to how you regularly communicate with the people you love. If you wouldn't talk that way to a co-worker or your boss, your family members certainly don't deserve it either.

Instead of taking out your frustrations on those closest to you, choose a healthier outlet: a bit of exercise, a talk with a friend or counselor, a power nap.

Exercise patience and understanding and find a direct path to more kindness, harmony and cooperation on the home front.

## Kindness and Happiness

There are scientific reasons for pumping up your kindness muscles. Research shows kindness makes us happier. People who perform random acts of kindness report being happier, and when the acts are varied – holding the door open for a stranger, helping someone with directions, doing a roommate's dishes – those happy feelings last longer than if you were to perform one act of kindness repeatedly.

## Kindness and Health

Beyond the happy feelings kindness brings, it is also good for your health. In his book *Meaning and Medicine,* Dr. Larry Dossey notes that kindness that you give, kindness that you receive, and even kindness that you observe from afar promotes a release of positive endorphins that Dossey termed *the helper's high.*

Allan Luks and Peggy Payne write extensively on the health benefits of kindness in their book *The Healing Power of Doing Good.*

In their extensive research they noted that those who regularly help people have a more optimistic and happier outlook on life. They report feeling more connected to people and have a higher sense of wellbeing.

They tend to have better immune systems, reduction of high blood pressure, improved circulation, reduced coronary disease, and no surprise, more energy. The benefits of kindness are endless, so what are you waiting for?

## Energizing Kindness

Begin your own kindness campaign by engaging in one small intentional act of kindness every day. I believe that kindness can be spread in meaningful ways every day and it needn't cost too much time or any money.

Start each day with openness to kindness. When you choose to walk with your head up and eyes open to the possibility of helping others, it's amazing what you will see.

We're living in a society that is immune to kindness in many ways and a simple *hello* might be met with a confused glance, but persevere. You never know when the smile or helping hand that you extend could turn someone's day around. It might be you that gets the boost.

I recall a day last spring when I was out for a run. I admit I was in a foul mood. I was tired and stressed out, and it seemed like nothing had gone right that day. I reluctantly dragged my butt out for some exercise in the hopes of feeling better.

It was a gorgeous, sunny day and I really had no reason to be in such a state, but there I was. Glass totally empty. As I ran through the park near my house I couldn't seem to find my mojo despite the fresh air and beauty that surrounded me. *Will this stupid run ever be over? Hmph.*

As I halfheartedly trudged onward I noticed a slightly slouched, diminutive old man shuffling along the path toward me. He wore a cardigan sweater buttoned neatly to the top and an old-style hat with a brim. He seemed unaware of me until I was within ten feet of him and then he simply stopped and watched me approach as if

I were the most important part of his day.

I was still feeling grumpy and antisocial but I made eye contact and forced a smile, and as I did, he flashed a happy grin, gave me a wink, and tipped his hat to me before continuing on his way. No words were exchanged, just a two-second connection that had the power to pull me out of my funk and back into a positive frame of mind. Ah, the power of a smile.

Connect with people. Look for chances to engage and assist. Say *thank you* more often. If you're thinking a kind thought about someone, take the time to email, call or visit them and let them hear your thoughts.

One small kind act a day is good for your health! Check out the ideas at the end of this chapter and include kindness as another endless source of energy.

## CHARGE!

Elton John said it best. *Sorry seems to be the hardest part.* Sometimes it's tough to admit when we're wrong. We tend to view an apology as a sign of weakness when in fact it requires great strength.

Forgiveness is a necessary path to energizing kindness. Do you have anyone in your life that you owe an apology to? You can tie up a lot of energy in a misunderstanding or grievance so set your energy free by making it right.

Below are four steps to help you with a simple heartfelt apology.

1. Let them know exactly what you're apologizing for.

2. Acknowledge how your actions impacted them. This validates their feelings and helps them see that you understand.

3. Take responsibility for the part you played without offering excuses or a story of defense.

4. Extend a genuine apology and ask for forgiveness.

Hugs and kisses all around!

## Whatever It Takes (*Positive Tickets*)

Here's a creative look at fostering kindness in youth. In 2001 the police force in Richmond, British Columbia, Canada, created the Positive Ticket Program to strengthen the relationship between police officers and Richmond's youth, and to reward kids for staying out of trouble.

Superintendent Ward Clapham calls it *catching kids being good*. He says his early years with the police led him to think he was doing too little, too late. Kids thought of police as the enemy, the people who arrested their parents. His idea was to start developing relationships that might keep kids from ever getting into trouble, to expand the focus of policing beyond just reacting to trouble.

Positive Tickets grew out of this idea, and in Richmond, officers now give out 50,000 tickets a year to kids they catch *doing the right thing*. The result has been a 41-percent drop in youth crime. In Richmond that represents 1,056 young people a year who never enter the criminal justice system.

By combining the efforts of the city and the police force, youth receive Positive Tickets for acts like wearing a bike helmet, not smoking, getting to school on time, helping out with a group of younger children, playing without causing a disturbance, and so on.

Kids redeem their tickets for activities that get them out into the community in a positive way. Thanks to partnerships with the City of Richmond and community businesses, ticketed kids can go swimming, skating, or even to a major sporting event, for free.

These days when kids in Richmond spot a patrol car they run toward it, not away. What a great idea. For more information on the Positive Ticket initiative visit *www.positivetickets.com*.

---

## ENERGY NOW!

---

### Please Be Kind

- Smile at a stranger, for no other reason than to be nice. That little gesture could turn their day around.
- Donate used books to a library.
- Volunteer at your local shelter, seniors' home, food bank or school.

- Why not do a job like mowing the lawn, cleaning the house or babysitting for someone, and surprise him or her by not charging?
- How good does it feel when someone you don't know compliments you on something? Do the same, and pass a genuine compliment on to a stranger.
- Start a piggy bank for a cause. Throw in spare change for one year and see how much you save!
- Bring music, conversation or reading to the elderly.
- Make a *random acts of kindness* list and be intentional in using it.
- Hold the door for someone.
- Reading together can be a very relaxing way to bond with a child you care about.
- Return your shopping cart instead of leaving it in the lot.
- Learn and remember the names of people you interact with often. Your dresser, dry cleaner, barista or mail carrier will feel recognized and appreciated.
- Write a letter to someone who has made a difference in your life.
- Talk with a homeless person. They are real people who have fallen on hard times.
- Pick up trash in your neighborhood, a park, or just on the street.
- Ask if you can help…anyone.
- Be kind to someone who is having a horrible day, even if they're not your favorite person.
- Say *I love you* more often.
- Smile more.
- Slow down and offer someone directions if they look lost.
- Leave a generous tip when you get great service.
- Say *good morning, thank you*, and *have a great day* as often as you can.
- Be a welcoming neighbor, a friend who listens and a co-worker who helps.
- Donate blood, used clothing, canned goods or your time.
- Be as nice to your family members as you are to co-workers, friends, neighbors and strangers.

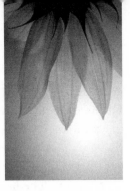

CHAPTER 12

# The Passion Project

*Chase down your passion like it's the last bus of the night.*
—TERRI GUILLEMETS

IN the year 2001 I developed a presentation entitled *But I've Never Climbed Everest?!* about overcoming small thinking and finding your passionate path through life. I created it out of frustration more than anything. My burning passion at the time was speaking in front of audiences and I wanted to grow that passion, but my deep-seated belief was that I hadn't done anything worthy of sharing with other people on a grand scale, that I didn't have a message worthy of keynote speaking.

I envied the Olympians, world adventurers and Everest summiteers who had done something *truly* remarkable with their lives.

The summer of 2000 I had seen adventurer Jeff Salz speak about his exploits climbing K2 and crossing the Arabian Desert, and that same year I also saw Jamie Clarke speak about his attempts to summit Everest. They were both empowering speakers and really had something interesting and adventurous to speak about. I wanted to be a keynote speaker too *But I've Never Climbed Everest.*

Passion has a powerful energy though. If you allow the voices to speak to you and let the dream in, ultimately it just rises to the surface. It can't help it.

It was while listening to another speaker at a conference later that same year that I had my epiphany. I'll be honest, I don't remember the conference and I don't remember the speaker, all I remember is that she had done some amazing things in her career as a track athlete, but she was a really lousy speaker: tedious, ultra-focused on herself, boring and uninspiring. That's ninety minutes of my life I'll never get back.

It wasn't a total loss though. In that mind-numbing hour and a half I did gain some valuable perspective. I sat there thinking, *I'm a good speaker. I can captivate and motivate an audience and it's not about what I've accomplished in my life, it's about how I can help my audiences accomplish more in theirs. That is my Everest. My passion is to help people and the speaking I so love is my vehicle to accomplish that in a bigger way.*

I began crafting the *Everest* presentation when I got home after that weekend – six steps to finding your passionate path, your *own* Everest, as it were. I've been helping people do just that for the last decade.

### pas·sion *noun*
**1** strong, barely controllable emotion.
**2** intense love or desire. **3** strong enthusiasm.

I hope you agree that passion is an essential ingredient in an energetic life. Just think about how energized you feel when you're doing something that you love. You'll get up early to do it, you'll pursue it for hours, you'll stay up late and not feel tired, you'll think about it when you're not doing it and still want more.

In my household, if our weekend plans include mountain biking or skiing it's so much easier to wake up early and burst out the door than when we're cleaning the garage or doing housework.

You know what I'm talking about. Reflect on the last time you were stuck doing something that you disliked immensely or that bored you silly: a lengthy meeting, the dentist, paying bills, studying. Not only does time seem to stand still in these situations, but your energy drains more quickly than water from a bathtub.

And I don't know about you, but the time drags on even more as I think about all the passion-filled pursuits I'd rather be doing.

## THE ENERGY CONNECTION

Passion is connected to purpose and without it life becomes routine, predictable and dull. There is energy in doing something meaningful in your life that you truly enjoy.

Your passion can be something as simple and comforting as needle-work or gardening. It can be as grand as starting a new business, changing your career, or changing the world. It can be physical or adventurous like mountain biking or paragliding. It can be connected to food, travel, art or music. If it puts a sparkle in your eye and a glow in your cheek – if you're passionate about it – it counts.

So, what are you passionate about? What puts a fire in your belly or brings you great joy and excitement? If you already know the answer to those questions ask yourself, *Am I regularly spending time in pursuit of my passion?* Are you?

When life gets busy we neglect our health by skipping exercise, eating less healthfully and sleeping less, but we also stop doing the things that we love with the mistaken belief that we can't afford to be frivolous with our time on *things like that.* You can't afford not to.

When you regularly spend time doing things that you love you just feel better, don't you? Passion feeds your spirit; it nurtures your self esteem and self-worth, which in turn improves your personal energy.

If you know what you're passionate about and you're not pursuing it, can you change that? Change it with the goal to have a bit more fun in your life, to make yourself more interesting to you, to live a more energetic life. Call it the passion project and start today.

Write down all the things that you love to do – big, small, and everything in between. Devote at least one hour each week to something on that list. If you're short on time try ten minutes per day.

Observe how you feel when you're in pursuit of your passions.

## FIND YOUR OWN EVEREST

*There is no end. There is no beginning.*
*There is only the passion of life.*
—FEDERICO FELLINI

*But what if I don't know what I'm passionate about?* This question is more common than you might think. Life has a way of stepping in the path of our passions until we forget we ever had any.

Work, childcare, family commitments, caring for aging parents, working more, taking care of household duties, struggling with finances, health, relationships, diapers, duties – life. One day you look up and can't remember the last time you did something truly for you. *I wouldn't know passion if it hit me in the face!*

So let me ask you a question. What gets you fired up? What gets you excited about getting out of bed and getting on with your day? I want you to really think about that. If there were no barriers in your way, what great and exciting things would you do with your life? It's a big question but it's a good starting point for finding your own Everest.

As a first step, grab a piece of paper and start writing down answers to that question. Ask yourself:

*What one great dream would I dare to*
*dream if I knew I could not fail?*

That means censorship buttons are off. Time and energy are abundant; you've got support from family and friends; money is not an issue; childcare is taken care of; you've got the education and experience you need; so really, you can do whatever your heart desires. What will it be? Write it down.

When you do this you will likely have one of two reactions. You may say to yourself *Just one? I have several great dreams,* or you will have trouble coming up with even one answer. If this second scenario sounds familiar, this next section is for you.

## SIX STEPS TO FINDING YOUR OWN EVEREST

It's time for a little more self-reflection and passion action. I hope you're up for it because there are few things on the planet more rewarding than connecting to your passion in a bigger more meaningful way.

### STEP 1. Come On, Get Happy

When I work through this exercise with my audiences the first question I ask them is, *Are you happy?* If you've read Chapter 10 then you know the impact of happiness on your energy. It's a good question to ponder as you move toward a more fulfilling, passion-filled life.

Most of us can hopefully look at our lives and answer a general *yes* to the question, so I want you to consider if there are any specific parts of your life that make you *unhappy.*

The unhappy parts of our lives pull energy away from growth opportunities and often cloud our judgement about what we're truly capable of. You can't ignore the things that make you unhappy and expect them to go away.

No matter the size of your unhappiness, it's worth working through for the energy you'll gain down the road. Identify your sources of sadness or stress and do whatever it takes to remove them from your life. Don't worry how long it will take, just start the ball rolling and continue on with step 2 of this passion project.

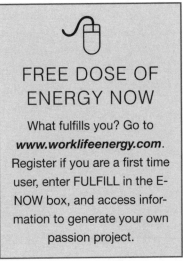

**FREE DOSE OF ENERGY NOW**

What fulfills you? Go to *www.worklifeenergy.com*. Register if you are a first time user, enter FULFILL in the E-NOW box, and access information to generate your own passion project.

### STEP 2. Spend More Time with Yourself

It will be near impossible to hone in on your passions if you're so caught up in daily tasks and doing for others that you don't take time for yourself.

Inspiration comes to us in moments of silence and reflection when the mind is calm enough to let new ideas in.

Spend some time with yourself. Sit in silent meditation in a place that brings you peace. That may be behind a closed bedroom door or in a hot bath. It could be in nature or at your favorite coffee shop.

Go for a walk alone or do some other activity that you enjoy and allow the exercise to act as a moving meditation. Let your mind flow around the sorts of things that bring you passion.

Reflect on things you used to do that brought you joy and fulfillment. Write them down and think about how they made you feel.

Ponder the activities you plan to take on when you have more time and energy in your life. What is it about those things that excite you? Ask yourself, *Why aren't I doing them now?*

Identify passions you'd like to push into the present and take small steps to integrate them into your life.

## STEP 3. Do a *Feel Good* Analysis

If you take the time to reflect on what you're passionate about and aren't hit with a wave of inspiration, fear not. What we want for ourselves changes over time, and you may be in a gap that needs a little extra attention.

As you go through your day, pay attention to what you currently do and what you're currently good at in your work and home life to get to what I call your *energy source*.

I'm sure there is a long list of things that you are good at. Maybe you're a whiz with computers or you're an amazing cook or baker. Perhaps you've got unbelievable skills with organizing or planning? It could be you have an affinity for languages, dance or athletics, or you can solve puzzles with speed and efficiency.

Often when a skill comes easily to us, we undermine its importance in the grand scheme. It doesn't occur to us that others may not execute these skills with the same ease as we do, so we dismiss them as ordinary. I'm certain if you really pay attention to everything that you're good at you'll realize you're far from ordinary.

A past audience member, Deidre, shared her *feel good* awareness with me after one of my talks. Several years earlier she was out at a pub with friends and had an epiphany while gyrating and bouncing around on the dance floor.

She realized that when she was dancing she felt truly alive. There was something about the movement and freedom of expression that woke something up in her so she decided to investigate that and signed up for a dance class at a local studio.

She wasn't surprised to learn that she loved dancing as much, if not more, when it wasn't accompanied by pints of beer. That first class lead to several more – hip hop, jazz, tap, even ballet – until several years later she found herself teaching dance classes part-time to young kids and teens.

She told me her full-time job as an accountant fed her responsible practical side and the dance classes fed her passion, plus she got great exercise.

Do you have anything like that in your life, perhaps hiding in plain sight? Remember that the pursuit of passion needn't be an all-or-nothing proposition and it doesn't need to be associated with paid work. It can simply be part-time energizing fun.

## STEP 4. Try New Things

If you've made it this far and you're still not finding your passion, maybe it's time to step out of the box and try something new, something you've never done before. Yes, it can be scary to venture into the unknown but it can also be very exhilarating.

I was in the middle of one of my presentations talking about this very point when I realized it had been a long time since I had tried something new myself.

I made the decision that year to train for a triathlon. I had always shied away from the challenge because I don't love swimming, or at least that's what I told myself. I had no problem with the running and cycling portions of the training, but in order to comfortably swim the 750-meter distance required of the sprint triathlon, I needed to get in the pool and practice.

As an athletic, fitness-oriented individual who teaches cycle classes and has tried dozens of different activities, I was surprised at how nervous I was the first time I ventured to the pool. You see, I didn't know *the rules*.

I wasn't sure of where to leave my towel or if I should take a water bottle with me to the pool deck. I didn't know if I could wear my flip flops as I walked to the pool from the changing room. I had no idea how fast of a swimmer I was, which lane I should be in, or what would happen if I had to take a rest at one end of the pool.

Small uncertainties like these can mean the difference between giving it a shot and giving up before you start. And since I wasn't even sure I liked swimming it all seemed like too much work, but I persevered.

I not only gained answers to all of my questions but I found out I'm a better swimmer than I thought I was, and learned that I loved the meditative nature of swimming lengths. It added a calming element to my usually frenetic, high-intensity exercise routine.

When you try new things you learn to overcome fears. The more small fears you overcome, the more empowered you will be to take on bigger challenges.

When you try new things you also get exposed to new experiences that will help you identify or eliminate potential passions.

One of my fellow life coaches learned through a very circuitous route that she loves (and I mean *loves*) hot yoga. Through a series of trials and errors, Carrie already knew that she wasn't much into traditional fitness classes, but she knew she needed a group fitness environment to keep her motivated.

In the quest for peace of mind and better fitness she thought she would try a Pilates class. The workout was challenging enough, but she wasn't able to *get in the groove* with the random exercises. Next she tried Ashtanga yoga, which she definitely preferred over Pilates. In that yoga class she complained to a friend that she felt like her muscles took forever to loosen up, and that's when she was introduced to the harmony of hot yoga.

A warm studio that soothes her stiff muscles combined with a predictable series of yoga postures that allows her to shut off her brain. Perfection. When Carrie describes hot yoga you can feel her passion. In that frame of mind she could sell ice to an Eskimo. Oops, wrong end of the thermometer.

I once took a series of watercolor art classes that helped me realize

I'm better off writing, or gardening, or painting walls, all of which I prefer tenfold to watercolor painting.

When you try new things it's as much about learning what you don't like as what you do. It will help direct you to new and wondrous possibilities.

## STEP 5. Learn to Break the Rules

I hope by now you've stumbled upon some sort of activity or passion that excites you enough to want to spend more time doing it.

The next step is about manifesting that passion in your life in a bigger way. The pursuit of your passions does not need to involve full-time, total immersion – but it could.

In 2005 I walked away from my safe and secure job in the fitness industry to launch my speaking business full time. Several years before that my partner left a high-profile, high-paying job in the oil and gas industry to pursue his passion for photography. Both leaps were scary and exciting and neither of us has looked back.

Until we made the leap though, you can bet there was some soul searching that took place, some barriers to knock down, and some questions to find answers to. If you know you want to pursue your passions in a bigger way, what's stopping you?

There is a wonderful quote in a novel called *Benjamin's Gift* that speaks to knocking down barriers that stand between you and your passions.

---

*He was convinced that laws existed only to guide the dull and the foolish and that a wise man's pleasure consisted in carefully and creatively subverting them.*
—MICHAEL GOLDING

---

If you want something badly enough, do whatever you need to do to make it happen. If it's important enough to you then any barrier is surmountable.

If you really want to live the dream, hatch a plan to bring it to reality. There is nothing more satisfying than getting up each day and doing a job that you love.

Oh, it has its highs and lows just like any other J.O.B., but when your work is connected to your passions the highs are sky-high and the lows are mere dips.

Regardless of whether you pursue your passions as a career or a hobby, the point is to pursue them. You'll add a richness and energy to your life that no amount of healthy food and sleep can match. Did I just say that? I think I did.

## STEP 6. Be S.M.A.R.T. About Your Passions

I was never a big fan of S.M.A.R.T. goals until I took my life coaching certification and learned a passion-driven form of goal setting that changed that for me.

The standard acronym for goal setting always felt too confined and safe to me. Specific and measurable I could grasp, but achievable, realistic and timely? Those guidelines don't feel very passion-filled, and why set a goal if it doesn't excite you?

In my life, most of my big lessons have come from setting big goals, maybe even unrealistic ones, that I had a good chance of *not* attaining.

For years I fantasized about being on *Oprah*, and while that was a significant stretch goal that never came to pass, it led me to conduct myself in a way that was congruent with an eventual guest spot on her show. What was there to lose? The TV show is now off the air, but hey, maybe I'll be on her radio show!

I've also learned a great deal about myself and my goals by connecting them to my passions. Making a career out of speaking with very little savings and even less of a plan may not have been the most realistic or achievable undertaking at the time, but I sure worked hard at it. I found success against the odds because I had skill as a speaker and was passionate about my goals.

I am a Co-Active Life Coach with the Coaches Training Institute (CTI) and when I was gaining my certification I was introduced to goal setting the CTI way.

Goals are meant to stretch you a little bit. They're meant to point you in the direction of your dreams and make you want to chase after them at all costs. You can't reach your goals unless you take action, and you won't take action on goals that don't excite you.

## Specific

Good goals are crystal clear in their outcome. What do you want for yourself? *I want to write a book someday* doesn't clarify my goal all that much. *I want to write a self-help book* gets a little clearer. If I say *I want to write a book to help people get more energy in their lives* it's easier to visualize the outcome and get started.

## Measurable

Make your goal measurable and attach a date to it. This step is essential because it helps you know when you're there.

If you want to reduce your credit card debt you can set a goal to pay off $1500 by February 15th. On that date you'll know whether you succeeded or not.

You might also set a goal to lose ten pounds by April 1st, or have five website pages built by October 30th. All are goals you can measure easily once the date arrives.

You've either reached the goal or you haven't. *By May 1st I will finish writing my thirteen-chapter book that will help people get more energy in their lives* is both measurable and specific.

## Accountable

This third step is where we depart from smart goals of old. Any goal worth making is worth moving toward in some meaningful way, so why not have someone hold you accountable to your process? I know what you're thinking: *The last thing I need is someone scolding me if I don't succeed.*

Accountability shouldn't be about guilt or nagging, it should be about support and focus. When I was writing the book proposal and first chapters for this book I met weekly via phone conference with two other authors and our book coach to talk about progress and set step-wise goals toward completion. They held me accountable to the process. At the late stages of book writing my publisher and my life coach both have a hand in that.

In the old model of goal setting I could tell myself that a fourteen-chapter book on personal energy was absolutely achievable – in fact I did...several times – but it wasn't until I connected accountability to my process that I *achieved* this ten-year-old goal. It's powerful stuff.

## Resonant

It's in these last two descriptions that goal setting becomes truly exciting. When you establish your own goals it might be worthwhile to start at these two steps and hone in on *specific* and *measurable* once you're clear (and excited) about what you want.

In this model we move away from *realistic* and replace it with *resonant*. What a great word.

**res·o·nant** *adj.*
a. Strong and deep in tone; resounding.
b. Having a lasting presence or effect; enduring.
c. Strongly reminiscent; evocative.

Is the goal you've set something you truly want? Does it move you toward the person you want to be? Does it have a *lasting presence* in your head and heart as you move toward completion?

If your goals don't resonate with you at a deeper level they will be harder to stay connected to. I always knew I wanted to write a book but I was rarely clear on the topic.

It was through some trial and error and a whole bunch of digging deep that I tapped into this idea of *energy now* that allows me to speak to all of the health and wellness ideas and philosophies I'm passionate about.

## Thrilling

Setting realistic goals might help you achieve them more easily but it likely won't help you grow beyond what you already know. *Timely* goals are safe. *Thrilling* goals are goals that you can't wait to get started on. If you've really found a goal that resonates with you, then work hard at this last step so you can experience the thrill of growth.

> *Set goals not for the accomplishment of the objectives,*
> *but for who you will become in accomplishing them.*
> —JIM RHONE

Your goal isn't meant to be something you feel you *should* do. Create a goal that inspires you and thrills you. Ask yourself, *What possibilities exist for me beyond my goal? What will its completion bring to my life? How will I feel?* Connect to that vision and get on with it. The world needs more movers and shakers like you.

Wouldn't you agree that *smart* goals established in this way are far more powerful than *achievable, realistic* and *timely* goals? The truth is, when we connect our goals to our passions it adds a power and presence to them that is difficult to ignore.

I'm proud to be a coach with CTI. If you're interested in learning more about the power of Co-Active Coaching, visit *www.thecoaches.com* to find your own coach or learn about becoming a coach yourself.

I know that once you recharge the passions in your life you will find a way to get to them regardless of how tired or busy you may feel right now. But should you find yourself feeling discouraged about that or any aspect of this energy-generating process, remind yourself that one small step is better than a thousand big thoughts.

Action is the answer. One small step today, another tomorrow, another the day after that, and you're back on track.

Isn't this fun?

## CHARGE!

Can you believe it? We're down to our last chapters. I hope that along with the page-turning you've also managed to implement a few small steps toward the changes you want and deserve for yourself.

I just said it: action is the answer. That's my simple wish for you at the end of this chapter – at the end of this book, really. Take action with your life, your health, your energy.

Visit *www.worklifeenergy.com* and enter the keywords I've shared with you throughout the book. Gain even more helpful information to guide you on this journey back to energy.

Ask for help via a life coach of your own, a friend, your church, your teachers or your family.

Get clear on what you really want for yourself and step into your new and energetic life.

## WHATEVER IT TAKES

I'm passionate about speaking, I'm passionate about helping people, and I'm passionate about having a bit of fun. Last year I decided to combine all three of those passions into a passion project of my own. I call it *The Clown Nose Project* and it started from a suggestion by an audience member.

In one of my presentations I share a story about taking life too seriously and how with the help of my twin sister, Christine, I learned to lighten up. My enlightenment involved clown noses that my sister, a drama teacher, was carrying in her vehicle.

I act out the scenario and use my red foam clown nose to help create the atmosphere. It's really quite funny.

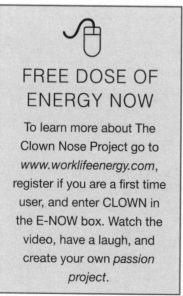

**FREE DOSE OF ENERGY NOW**

To learn more about The Clown Nose Project go to *www.worklifeenergy.com*, register if you are a first time user, and enter CLOWN in the E-NOW box. Watch the video, have a laugh, and create your own *passion project*.

At the end of one of those presentations an audience member suggested that I sell clown noses at my events. I agreed that it would be fun but wondered if it was worth all the effort for the small profit I would make on each sale. But maybe it didn't have to be about what *I* could gain from it; clown noses are fun. If I could make the sale of them meaningful somehow, I could probably sell a lot of noses.

I recalled that for many years fitness colleagues Alan and Jackie ran a very successful *Twoonie Yoga* class in my city. They charged just $2 to attend the Sunday morning class. They shared the magic of yoga with a loyal following and donated all the proceeds to local charities. *Twoonie Yoga* started in September of 2002 and to date they have raised over $40,000.00 and helped ten charities, two dollars at a time. It's an accomplishment they can really be proud of.

I thought *I can do that!* In October of 2010 I started *The Clown Nose Project* to raise money for various charities through the sale of clown noses.

For $2 my audience members get to experience the joy and silliness of wearing a clown nose with their co-workers or kids, and I get the pleasure of helping an organization in need.

My project is in its infancy but it has a lot of energy and we're well on the way to making a difference for one special organization, one clown nose at a time.

## ENERGY NOW!

### Recharge Your Passions

- Do one thing every day that excites and thrills you.
- Think out-of-the-box about new experiences. Plan outings that spark your interests in unique ways.
- Create a thrilling, resonant goal and see how it feels.
- Try something new.
- Reconnect with something you used to enjoy doing.
- Don't take no for an answer.
- Talk to someone who inspires you that is doing work you're interested in.
- Instead of saying It can't be done, reframe to How can I make it happen?
- Join a club that does what you love – cycling, dance, books, art, science, stamp-collecting…
- Write down ten things you love to do. Post them where you can view them daily. Do one tomorrow.

- Schedule in a monthly passion project that helps you get closer to a valued goal.
- Take time for yourself to do something just for you.
- Volunteer with an organization in line with your passions.
- Feel the fear and do it anyway.
- Surround yourself with people who embrace life fully. Uninspired people are…well…
- What makes your heart sing? Whatever it is, do more of that.
- Life is meant to be LIVED. Connect with people and experiences you're passionate about.
- Read books about things you dream of doing. Education elicits action.
- Create a vision board with pictures and words that inspire you on your path to greatness.
- Passion is about filling your heart with love…for anything. I'm passionate about my dog!
- I'm passionate about good food, fitness, and life balance too. Define yours and live it.
- Kiss, kiss. Hug, hug. That kind of passion matters too. Who do you love? Show them just how much.
- When you were a kid, what excited you? Tree climbing? Lego? Fishing? Play with that today.
- Connect with people who are doing good in the world. Passion is contagious.
- Talk to people who love their work. Ask them what makes that happen and do it too.
- Walking away from something you don't love is akin to walking toward wondrous possibilities. That ain't failure, baby.

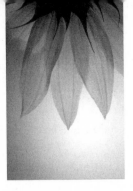

CHAPTER 13

# Small Steps to an Energetic Life

*It is better to take many small steps in the right direction
than to make a great leap forward only to stumble backward.*
—CHINESE PROVERB

Y OU'VE got the concept: small steps to great gains. You have
some idea in your head about what you'd like to accomplish
for yourself. So if you haven't done so already, how about
you get started? Take a few energy-producing steps with some of
the ideas you've read.

If fatigue, lack of time, and low motivation are still getting in the
way, know that your energy will improve at a remarkable rate once
you take the first step.

Recognize the enemy. Temptation will present as food cravings
or your comfy armchair, procrastination will disguise itself as misplaced
sneakers, the television and internet will always be there to distract you.

Excuses will pop up when someone needs your attention now,
when *anything* needs your attention now or distracts you away from
your ultimate goal of self-care.

When energy and motivation are low, the excuse that gets you off track doesn't need to be big. It might be only slightly less agreeable than whatever you're avoiding and that will be enough to sidetrack your efforts.

Case in point, when I'm doing something enjoyable I could care less if my floor is swept or the laundry is done, but if I have something undesirable on my to-do list I have the cleanest house on the block. Compared to organizing receipts for my bookkeeper I *love* cleaning the toilets!

Tackle temptation, push past procrastination, destroy those distractions and ignore the excuses.

You can do this. You know that anything good that happens in your life, any goal that you achieve, or any barrier that you knock down that's in the way of your success happens because you make it happen.

Your life really is up to you. Good, bad or average. So why not choose good? Good. Now let's increase our chances of getting this right!

## Believe You Can Achieve Your Plan

The following ideas will help you get moving and keep you going when time and energy are talking you out of action. They will remind you that you are truly able to accomplish anything you set your mind to if you only believe it.

> *Rule # 1: Use your good judgment in all situations.*
> *Rule #2: There are no additional rules.*
> —Anonymous

### Decide That You're Worth It

After all you've read I hope your good judgment is pushing you toward change. You're worth it. But in a busy life with so much on your plate it can be difficult to accept, so I want to make sure you're convinced. I have two tough cases to share that may help.

## CASE #1

Mark, a personal training client, was having a difficult time prioritizing his fitness. He told me he really didn't have time to exercise regularly because he had three sons who were involved in so many activities that needed his time.

If he wasn't driving his oldest to karate class he was dropping off or picking up one of his younger sons at hockey or soccer, or watching from the sidelines. He worked all day and felt after-work time should be for them. Stuck between a rock and a hard place he said, *They need me! What kind of father chooses to exercise instead of being at his kids sporting events?*

He had a point…to a point. You see he had gained thirty pounds and lost his own health just so his kids could keep theirs. While he was indeed a supportive and loving father, he certainly wasn't a role model for health and fitness.

## CASE #2

Several years ago while presenting at a day-long wellness conference I had a chat with a woman named Tracy who admitted to me that she felt guilty doing indulgent things for herself.

She felt guilty for being at the event, she felt guilty taking time away from home responsibilities to go exercise or spend time with friends, she felt unworthy of praise bestowed upon her, and when it came right down to it she didn't believe she was worth any of it.

She was at a beautiful hotel in the Canadian Rockies where we were being treated to wonderful food, inspiration and fun and she couldn't allow herself to simply enjoy it.

Mark and Tracy both had everyone else's needs and best interests on their mind all the time and had forgotten how to prioritize themselves. It's not an uncommon occurrence, is it?

Yes, when life gets busy and the to-do list is long, it is too easy to put everyone and everything else before your own needs.

Reality check: if you keep it up for too long you'll burn out and have nothing left to give anybody. It's why you picked up this book in the first place, isn't it?

*You yourself, as much as anybody in the entire*
*universe, deserve your love and affection.*
—BUDDHA

It's time to take care of you. Put yourself back on your priority list once and for all. Too difficult, you say?

Do it anyway, if only to stay fuelled up and energized for your continued life of martyrdom. Decide that you're worth a little selfish self-care if only so you can continue to give unselfishly to everyone and everything else. Wait, I have a better idea...

Do it for you. Make a decision right now to do whatever it takes to generate more energy, experience greater health, and recharge your life just the way you'd like.

Decide that a little time devoted to yourself is a good investment in your own needs. Do something great for yourself *just because*. Become a more interesting, healthier version of yourself just for you.

## Establish Your First Goal

Once you've decided you're worth spending a little time on, it can be appealing to jump in with all you've got. I know you're excited about the new and improved version of you that waits just around the next corner, but I have to caution you from going too big right out of the gate. Isn't that crazy?

You're charged up and I'm cutting your flow of energy. Well, I'm doing this for the following two important reasons.

## Too Much of a Good Thing

Any time you add something new to your daily routine there will be an adjustment period as your current responsibilities get shuffled into new positions.

If you add in exercise after work, all the tasks you usually do at that time need to find a new home. The grocery shopping will be delayed, arrangements need to be made to deal with school pick up, and dinner will be later than normal.

While you'll eventually adjust to the differences, it will feel awkward and unmanageable at first. Small steps allow for gradual habituation to the new behaviors and greater likelihood of imprinting these habits for the long term. Yay for you!

## Too Many Choices

If you vow to start exercising, revamp your eating, and quit smoking all at once the chances of stalling on all three are higher than succeeding at just one.

Establish the first goal to which you want to habituate. Commit to it at a higher level *and* continue to take small daily steps in the other areas.

For instance, if your first goal is to create a routine around your exercise, you have to decide which days, at what times, and what you'll do when you get to it.

Then you'll need to step into your new plan and see how it goes. As you habituate to the new routine your determination will be tested with those familiar time, energy and motivation challenges. Then what?

You'll need all of your energy and resolve to push through and keep to your plan. Imagine if you also had to do this with every meal choice or career goal too?

Instead, throw the bulk of your resolve on your first goal and continue with small daily efforts on the others. Once you've created a habit around goal number one, then you can step up your efforts on the next and the next.

Interestingly, as you begin to make better choices in one area those good feelings will overlap into other health and self-care decisions almost without effort.

## Tell Someone Your Plan

What is so difficult about going public with a plan for lifestyle change? Why might you be hesitant to tell your best friend you're starting an exercise program or diet? What is so hard about telling your spouse or partner that you've decided to quit smoking?

It's a simple exercise in self-preservation, really. By keeping these lifestyle change plans to ourselves, no one else needs to share the news if our efforts end in failure. And they often do when we employ this method because if you have no one to hold you accountable you won't work as hard to realize success.

Sure, silence gives you an easy way out but it doesn't bring you any closer to your goal. Why not challenge yourself a bit?

---

*It takes a lot of courage to show your dreams to someone else.*
—ERMA BOMBECK

---

The more people you tell, the more likely you are to work at your goal so you don't let them or yourself down. Tell at least one person about your plan.

*Tomorrow I am going to start my daily walking program. I want to walk fifteen to twenty minutes every day on my lunch break.*

Choose your support carefully, guide them on the type of support you need, and allow them to check in with you and hold you accountable for the plan you've set out to achieve.

*I'm telling you this because you seem to be successful with your own exercise routine and it might help me stay motivated. I don't need you to hover over me to make sure I keep at it but I wouldn't mind the occasional check-in. And maybe I could let you know if I'm struggling and need some support?*

Your accountability partner could be a family member or a good friend, but it could just as easily be a co-worker whom you interact with regularly or someone you see daily in your neighborhood.

It could be a member of your church community, your counselor, or a life coach.

And these days you can gain viable support via internet support groups or even social networking. Hey, find me on Twitter and we'll talk!

No matter the source, you'll be amazed at how motivating a little well-placed accountability can be.

## Take Small Steps

I don't want to belabor this small steps philosophy. Wait…actually, I do! Take small steps *every day* in key areas of your life where you want to improve – exercise, healthy eating, saving money, nurturing your relationship, relaxing, learning a new language, developing your business – and just imagine how much progress you will make 365 days from now.

---

*The secret to getting ahead is getting started.*
*The secret of getting started is breaking your complex,*
*overwhelming tasks into small manageable tasks,*
*and then starting on the first one.*
—MARK TWAIN

---

Small steps applied consistently over time are so much more effective than unrealized thoughts. Have I made my point clear yet? Take a small step toward your big goal every day. It isn't rocket science. If you take action there will be a payoff somewhere down the line. Don't think so much…do something!

This small steps model works with anything you want to be spending time at and you will increase your success through consistency.

## Do It Daily to Create a Habit

You know that thing you did yesterday toward your goal? Do it *again* today. I know you're tired, and maybe still celebrating what you accomplished yesterday. And you should be proud, but we're not doing things like we used to any more so get back to work. Step up your game. Celebrate what you did yesterday, then do it again today.

---

*Action will destroy your procrastination.*
—OG MANDINO

---

Begin creating the habits today that will bring you more energy and better health tomorrow. Do a little less if you need to but don't give in to old behaviors that would have you making excuses and skipping out on change. Consistency brings about familiarity and familiarity increases confidence. Once you start to believe in your capabilities there will be no stopping you. Start small and do it daily. Hey…and tomorrow reread this suggestion.

## Mark Your Progress

If you don't think those daily small steps will amount to much, then start writing them down. Nothing will bring more clarity to your actions than that.

There are two great ways you can write and record your thoughts and successes each day. The first is to create a daily self-care checklist so you're reminded to fit yourself into your schedule. Get yourself a journal and use it to set your intentions each morning.

Make a list that includes what you'll do for exercise, how you'll improve your eating, what to do for fun, career growth, rest and relaxation – even hydration. Whatever you want to improve upon, add it to the list. Just remember to keep the steps small so you can get to them in a day. Check out my *GOT TO IT* journal at *www.got-toit.ca* to see what I mean.

As you accomplish each small goal enjoy the satisfaction of checking them off your list. There's no better feeling, is there? No wonder! Research has shown that we experience a release of positive endorphins every time we get to do that. Maybe it's just a wee little endorphin rush but it beats the heck out of stressing that you're not getting anything done from your go-big-or-go-home task list!

At the end of the day take stock of your success. You set boundaries and put yourself back on your priority list. You did what you said you would.

Exercise, healthy eating, personal growth – these are things you're used to skipping, delaying and procrastinating over. Not anymore! And you feel pretty good about yourself when you're done, don't you? Hold on to that feeling. It gets better.

> *Balance is not better time management but*
> *better boundary management. Balance means*
> *making choices and enjoying those choices.*
> —BETSY JACOBSON

The second way you can mark your progress is to write down your thoughts around your new self-care process. You're changing your lifestyle one small step at a time. You will have experiences worth remembering, and come up against road blocks you'll need to figure a way past.

Ask yourself what's working. Write down things you've struggled with. Note how you're feeling each day. Vent your frustrations. Record your successes. The insights you gain through this process will be mind-boggling, I promise you!

Not much into writing? I say *tough luck*. Dare to do it differently this time, at least in the initial stages of your plan.

With so much new information and behaviors to sort through, you can't expect your memory to serve you perfectly as you navigate the highs and lows of this journey.

Try five minutes of journaling a day. Heck, even quick notes will serve to imprint the lessons as you go along. You'll get a kick out of rereading them somewhere down the line – perhaps in astonishment for all you've learned and accomplished since you launched this expedition back to energy.

## Buddy Up

You've already told someone your plans, so why not include them in what you're doing? Yup, misery indeed loves company, and initially that's what it may feel like, but after a while I'll bet you'll start to enjoy what you're doing simply because you have someone to share the highs and lows with.

> *Accountability breeds response-ability.*
> —STEPHEN COVEY

An exercise buddy will help you drag your butt off the sofa if only so you don't let them down. Believe me, they'll be feeling the same way toward you.

A healthy eating partner will commiserate with you when you're craving those french fries, and tell you all the reasons why they're worth skipping. In the next sentence your partner may tell you how they nearly lost it when walking past the bakery. It will feel good to work out your challenges together. I think that kind of support is worth something.

I used to indoor climb with a friend of mine through the winter and every week as I got into her vehicle we'd both start whining about how long the day had been, how cold it was outside and how tired we were…and *Maybe we should just go for a beer?*

Every week we'd engage in the same back-and-forth discussion about whether we should climb or go for a beer…go for a beer or climb…climb or go for a beer…and just like the week before (and the week before that…and the several weeks before *that*), after two minutes we'd talk each other into climbing. It was comical in its predictability, but that's the power of accountability.

Sometimes she was the strong one, sometimes I was, but you can bet that if either of us was making the decision alone we'd have climbed a lot less.

An accountability partner will be your best friend as you work toward a personal or professional goal that has previously met with procrastination. And when you're having those moments of feeling sorry for yourself, remember that sometimes a little suffering will be part of the game.

Just because it's something that you want – better health, a thriving business, a published book, a healthy bank account – doesn't mean you're going to be excited and motivated to get to it, but that doesn't mean it won't be worth every single *I'd rather be doing anything else* moment you suffer through on the path to completion.

As I write this chapter I'm on a three-hour flight and truthfully, I would rather be watching a movie, but I made a commitment to my writing group that I would produce two more chapters on this week of travel. So I write if only to avoid their scorn and my feelings of guilt. Frankly, it feels good to get to it!

## Troubleshoot Those Road Blocks

As you continue on your journey toward personal and professional energy and abundance you will stumble from time to time. There will be days when you'll want to run back to what you knew if only because it wasn't so much darn work. There will also be more good days than bad, and more victories than defeats.

> *Obstacles are those frightful things you see*
> *when you take your eyes off your goal.*
> —HENRY FORD

You can guide that process if you like. Look ahead in your schedule. Are there any days or weeks that may present challenges you should be aware of? If you're trying to lose weight, big parties or social events can disrupt your healthy-eating efforts. Take note and make a plan.

Will your work schedule get in the way of regular exercise somewhere down the line? Anticipate the busyness and make sure you fit in your fitness in small steps – no matter what.

Who are the people in your life who might try to get in the way of your success? Have a chat with them. Negotiate a plan that will help them support and not sabotage.

What will you do when fatigue and lack of time rear their ugly heads? They will, you know. They always have. Think about it now while you're enthusiastic for change. Write down your plan, post it where you can see it, and set yourself up for success once and for all.

## Build a Healthy Environment Around You

> *Be careful the environment you choose for it*
> *will shape you; be careful the friends you choose*
> *for you will become like them.*
> —W. CLEMENT STONE

Perhaps one of the biggest roadblocks you'll come up against in your change efforts will be the people around you and the places you frequent.

For instance, it's very difficult to embrace healthy, success-oriented choices if you're hanging out on the sofa or at the bar, surrounded by people who could care less about your success, or their own for that matter.

If you're trying to become more positive, steer clear of the negative people and naysayers, who couldn't see the good in a situation if it hit them in the face. If you're trying to save money it's probably best to avoid the people and places that prompt you to spend.

If you put yourself in the right environment with the right people, who are aligned with the goals you want for yourself, you'll find it's much easier to stumble over success.

When a friend of mine was trying to lose weight she had to make a conscious choice not to go for coffee with her regular work pals. They always went around the corner to a bakery that made these amazing, huge, icing-topped cupcakes that no longer fit with her new plan. Instead she began tagging along with two other co-workers who used their coffee break to take a walk.

Not only was she saving over 500 calories every day by skipping the cupcake, but she was burning calories on her daily walks and learning from two women who had figured out a few things she needed to learn about health and wellness. Talk about a healthy alliance!

If you surround yourself with competent, conscientious, and supportive people who exhibit the same sorts of behaviors you want in your own life, it can only rub off on you.

It's tough to consider that you may need to revise your circle of friends in order to increase your chances of success, but if they're not willing to join you on the journey and are bringing you down, then maybe it's time. Why should you accept less for yourself just because the people around you do?

Put yourself in the path of people who have figured it out. Surround yourself with positive, driven and supportive role models. Avoid haunts that tempt you into bad habits. Create an environment of support that will help you realize your goals and dreams sooner rather than later.

### Develop a *No-Matter-What* Mindset

The foundation is set. The rest is up to you. This time, instead of working at your new goals for a short spell and then throwing in the towel, tell yourself, *I'm doing it no matter what.*

How will anything change if you don't?

Believe me, you'll try and talk yourself out of it more times than you can imagine. Who wants to exercise when they're tired at the end of a long day? How much fun is fresh fruit when you could have cheesecake? And I'm sure organizing your office or writing that business plan is the last thing you want to do on a Saturday afternoon, but if not now, then when?

> *Don't let the fear of the time it will take to accomplish something stand in the way of your doing it. The time will pass anyway; we might just as well put that passing time to the best possible use.*
> —Earl Nightingale

Circumstances won't change unless you do. Dare to do it differently this time. Do it even when you don't want to. Do it just because you can!

And here's where the brilliance of small steps becomes very apparent: if every fiber in your body is talking you out of doing whatever it is you planned to do, stick with your *no-matter-what* plan and simply do *less*. Doing on a small level is so much better than thinking about going big. Your goal is accomplished for today. That's all there is to it.

## Celebrate Every Day!

I'm a fan of goal setting if only for the opportunity to achieve the outcome and celebrate success. You don't get to do that very often when goals are lofty and out-of-reach.

It's one of the benefits of my small-steps approach. You get to celebrate small successes every day as you consistently move toward the bigger goals and dreams that up until now sat idly waiting for you to find the time to go big.

Do you see what's happening here? If you keep at it in small steps every day you *will* reach your goals. No more sitting on the sofa feeling sorry for yourself because *nothing good ever happens to you*. Go out and make it happen.

> *When the world says, Give up,*
> *Hope whispers, Try it one more time.*
> —AUTHOR UNKNOWN

You're capable. Keep telling yourself that every day when you check off more completed items. Tell yourself *I Rock*. Celebrate consistent small steps and encourage yourself to keep moving. Oh it's happening all right!

## CHARGE!

I have nothing more to say to you except *Congratulations!* Congratulations for the effort you gave to reading this book. Congratulations for the good things you will do for your self-care starting now.

You're now armed with enough small-steps information to live an energetic life – mind, body and spirit – so don't wait another day. Get up and get on with it. CHARGE!

### WHATEVER IT TAKES

Remember Mark and Tracy from the start of this chapter? They both had unique challenges around putting themselves on their own priority list, and they both figured out a way through!

After much discussion and brainstorming Mark devised a plan to put his sideline time to double duty. When he was at the soccer field, instead of sitting with all the other spectators he began walking the sidelines – one end to the other – back and forth all game long.

At the hockey arena he climbed the stairs – up and down – for at least ten minutes every period. Not only did he get to watch the game from

**FREE DOSE OF ENERGY NOW**

To find out other ways that Michelle can energize your life, visit *www.worklifeenergy.com*, register if you *still* haven't visited, and enter NEWS in the E-NOW box. See what fun awaits.

varied vantage points, but he burned hundreds and hundreds of calories when normally he would be adding them on sipping hot chocolate and eating licorice like he used to do while he watched.

Over the weeks his energy soared and his weight plummeted, and Mark wasn't forced to take one moment away from being a good dad. Nice work, Mark!

Tracy was a tougher nut to crack. She realized that she undervalued herself and knew it likely had something to do with how she was raised. As the oldest child of four siblings she was always expected to help out, be responsible, take care of the younger kids, and since her parents were busy running a farm she rarely got the praise she deserved and more often than not it was the opposite.

She chose to see a counselor, which was probably the most self-indulgent (read: wonderful) thing she could do for herself, despite the guilt and fear she felt around it. Over time she talked her way out of her martyrdom and into new and wonderful experiences for herself. She told me a couple of years later that once she found herself and began doing *for* herself, her kids began treating her differently too – *with respect,* she told me with much surprise.

No surprise there! How about you? When was the last time you threw caution to the wind and put yourself at the top of your priority list?

Decide that a little time devoted to yourself is a good investment in your own needs. Become a more interesting, healthier version of yourself just for you. *Do whatever it takes.*

## ENERGY NOW!

### Stay on Track

- Start your day with one positive thought about YOU.
- Write it out and place it by your bed to remind you.
- Exchange negative thoughts with positive options twice today.
- Develop a personal growth mantra that resonates with you and is repeatable when motivation and enthusiasm begin to falter.

- Choose to disengage from office gossip.
- Smile at a total stranger.
- Smile at yourself in the mirror. Try to mean it.
- Create your AMAZING LIST: a list of twenty words that describe what's amazing about you. Read it once a day.
- Write down a long-desired goal and post it where you can simply look at it.
- Do one small thing on your self-care to-do list...right now.
- Think of one thing you've done lately that you're proud of. Revel in it for a moment.
- Write down three things you're grateful for before you sleep tonight.
- Do it again tomorrow night.
- You ROCK!

# REFERENCES

## Chapter 2. The Energy Now! Philosophy

Bohl, D. (2011). *A smarter approach to time management.* Retrieved from www.pickthebrain.com/blog/smarter-time-management.

Cederberg, M. (2009). *Got to It.* Calgary, AB: Live Out Loud Speaking and Consulting, Inc.

Day, S. (2011). *Eating the elephant: tackling big goals.* Retrieved from Sherry Day ezinearticles.com/?Eating-the-Elephant--Tackling-Big-Goals&id=3553708.

Heath, C, & Heath, D. (2010). *Switch: How to Change Things When Change Is Hard.* Toronto, ON: Random House.

Knaus, W. J. (1998). *Do It Now: Break the Procrastination Habit.* New York, NY: John Wiley & Sons.

Selkirk, D. (2009). *Catching kids being good.* Retrieved from www.shared-vision.com/svvisionaries/catching-kids-being-good.

Wikipedia. (2010, May 02). *Psychological hedonism.* Retrieved from en.wikipedia.org/wiki/Psychological_hedonism.

## Chapter 4. Taking Down the Time Bandits

Covey, S. (1994). *First Things First.* London: Simon & Schuster UK Ltd.

Nedd, K. (2004). *Power Over Stress: 35 Quick Prescriptions for Mastering the Stress in Your Life.* Toronto, ON: QP Press.

Pavelka, J. (2000). *It's Not About Time: Rediscovering Leisure in a Changing World.* Carp, ON: Creative Bound, Inc.

The Walking Golfer. (2011). *The physical benefits of walking when you golf.* Retrieved from www.thewalkinggolfer.com/ benefits_of_walking/physical.html.

Wilmore, J., Costil, D. & Kennedy, L. (2008). *Physiology of Sport and Exercise.* Champaign, Illinois: Human Kinetics Press.

## Chapter 5. Fitness: Exercise Less for Success

American College of Sports Medicine. (2007). *Physical activity and public health guidelines.* Retrieved from www.acsm.org/AM/ Template.cfm?Section=Home_Page&TEMPLATE=/ CM/HTMLDisplay.cfm&CONTENTID=7764.

Brooks, D. (2001). *Effective Strength Training.* Champaign, Illinois: Human Kinetics.

Dariush Mozaffarian, M.D., Dr. P.H., Tao Hao, M.P.H., Eric B. Rimm, Sc.D., Walter C. Willett, M.D., Dr. P.H., and Frank B. Hu, M.D., Ph. D. (2011). Changes in diet and lifestyle and long-term weight gain in women and men. *New England Journal of Medicine, 364*: 2392-2404.

Public Health Agency of Canada. (2011, January 01). *Physical activity: tips to get active.* Retrieved from www.phac-aspc.gc.ca/ hp-ps/hl-mvs/pa-ap/07paap-eng.ph.

Roizen, M, & Mehmet, C. (2005). *You: The Owner's Manual.* New York, NY: Harper Resource.

Sharkey, B. (1997). *Fitness and Health (4th ed.).* Champaign, Illinois: Human Kinetics.

U.S Department of Health and Human Services. (2009, November 04). *Physical activity guidelines for Americans.* Retrieved from www.health.gov/paguidelines/default.aspx.

## Chapter 6. Nutrition: Fuelling a New You One Bite at a Time

Albers, S. (2009). *50 Ways to Sooth Yourself Without Food.* Oakland, CA: New Harbinger Publications, Inc.

Bean, A. (2009). *The Complete Guide to Sports Nutrition.* London: A & C Black Publishers Ltd.

Clark, Nancy. (1997). *Nancy Clark's Sports Nutrition Guidebook.* Windsor, ON: Human Kinetics.

Diet.com. (2004). *Macronutrients.* Retrieved from www.diet.com/g/macronutrients.

Harvard School of Public health. (2011). *The bottom line: choose good carbs, not no carbs. whole grains are your best bet.* Retrieved from www.hsph.harvard.edu/nutritionsource/what-should-you-eat/carbohydrates/index.html.

Health Canada. (2011, March 07). *Eating well with Canada's food guide.* Retrieved from www.hc-sc.gc.ca/fn-an/food-guide-aliment/index-eng.php.

Helpguide.org. (2011). *Choosing healthy fats good fats, bad fats, and the power of omega-3 fats.* Retrieved from www.helpguide.org/life/healthy_diet_fats.htm.

Kleiner, S. (2007). *Power Eating: Build Muscle, Gain Energy, Lose Fat.* Champaign, IL: Human Kinetics.

Resch, E, & Tribole, E. (2009). *Intuitive Eating: A Practical Guide to Make Peace with Food, Free Yourself from Chronic Dieting, Reach your Natural Weight.* Louisville, CO: Sounds True.

United States Department of Agriculture. (2011, February 22). *My pyramid.org: Steps to a healthier you.* Retrieved from www.mypyramid.gov.

Web MD. (2011). *The skinny on fats: good fats vs. bad fats.* Retrieved from www.webmd.com/diet/features/skinny-fat-good-fats-bad-fats.

Welsh, J, Sharma, A, Abramson, J, Vaccarino, V, Gillespie, C., & Vos, M. (2010). Caloric sweetener consumption and dyslipidemia among us adults. *Journal of the American Medical Association, 303*(15), 1490-1497.

Willett, A. (2005). *Eat, Drink, and Be Healthy: The Harvard Medical School Guide to Healthy Eating.* New York, NY: Free Press.

Wikipedia . (2011, April 06). *Intuitive eating.* Retrieved from en.wikipedia.org/wiki/Intuitive_eating.

Whitmore, B, & Milkovich, L. (2005). *Vitality & Vitals.* Calgary, AB: Vitality and Vitals Inc.

## Nutrition Resources

Albers, S. (2009). *50 Ways to Sooth Yourself Without Food.* Oakland, CA: New Harbinger Publications, Inc.

Craving Change. (2008). *Craving Change: A How to Guide for People Who Struggle with Their Eating.* Retrieved from www.cravingchange.ca.

Resch, E, & Tribole, E. (2009). *Intuitive Eating: A Practical Guide to Make Peace with Food, Free Yourself from Chronic Dieting, Reach your Natural Weight.* Louisville, CO: Sounds True.

## Healthy Cookbooks

Podleski, J, & Podleski , G. (2005). *Eat, Shrink & Be Merry! Great-tasting Food that Won't Go from Your Lips to Your Hips.* Kitchener, ON: Granet Publishing. Inc.

Reno, T. (2009). *Tosca Reno's Eat Clean Cookbook: Delicious Recipes that Will Burn Fat and Re-shape Your Body!.* Mississauga, ON: Robert Kennedy Publishing.

Reno, T. (2010). *The Best of Clean Eating: Over 200 Mouthwatering Recipes to Keep You Lean and Healthy.* Mississauga, ON: Robert Kennedy Publishing.

Van Rosendaal, J. (2007). *One Smart Cookie: All Your Favourite Cookies, Squares, Brownies and Biscotti... with Less Fat.* Vancouver, BC: Whitecap Books.

## Chapter 7. Hydration: Water You Drinking?

Got Water. (2006). *Water tips.* Retrieved from www.gotwater.net/water_tips.htm.

Hooked on Juice. (2006, October 02). *Hooked on juice.* Retrieved from www.hookedonjuice.com/.

Quinn, E. (2011, April 15). *What to drink for proper hydration during exercise.* Retrieved from sportsmedicine.about.com/od/hydrationand-fluid/a/ProperHydration.htm.

Science Daily. (2010). *"Drink at least 8 glasses of water a day" – really?.* Retrieved from www.sciencedaily.com/releases/2002/08/020809071640.htm.

World health net. (2011). *Hydration.* Retrieved from www.world-health.net/news/hydration.

Chapter 8. Sleep. The Quest for Rest and Relaxation

Dement, W.C. (2000). *The Promise of Sleep: A Pioneer in Sleep Medicine Explores the Vital Connection Between Health, Happiness, and a Good Night's Sleep.* New York: Dell.

Epstein, L. & Mardon, S. (2007). *The Harvard Medical School Guide to a Good Night's Sleep.* New York, NY: McGraw-Hill.

Hauri, P. & Linde, S. (1996). *No More Sleepless Nights. Rev. Ed.* New York, NY: Wiley & Sons.

Mayo Clinic. (2010, November 05). *10 tips for better sleep.* Retrieved from www.mayoclinic.com/health/sleep/HQ01387.

National Sleep Foundation. (2011). *How much sleep do we really need?.* Retrieved from www.sleepfoundation.org/article/how-sleep-works/how-much-sleep-do-we-really-need.

Read, T. (2009). *Till Sex Do Us Part: Make Your Married Sex Irresistible.* Toronto: Key Porter Books.

## Chapter 9. Stress Less for Success

American Institute of Stress. (2010). *America's no. 1 health problem.* Retrieved from www.stress.org/americas.htm.

American Institute of Stress. (2010). *Stress, definition of stress, stressor, what is stress? eustress?.* Retrieved from www.stress.org/topic-definition-stress.htm.

American Heart Association. (2011). *Four ways to deal with stress.* Retrieved from www.heart.org/HEARTORG/GettingHealthy/StressManagement/FourWaystoDealWithStress/Four-Ways-to-Deal-with-Stress_UCM_307996_Article.jsp.

Helpguide.org. (2011). *Laughter is the best medicine the health benefits of humor and laughter.* Retrieved from www.helpguide.org/life/humor_laughter_health.htm.

Herring, J (2011). *Stress Management: Never Get Too Hungry, Angry, Lonely, Tired, or Scared.* Retrieved from ezinearticles.com/?Stress-Management:-Never-Get—Too-Hungry,-Angry,-Lonely,-Tired,-or-Scared&id=68757.

Nedd, K. (2004). *Power Over Stress: 35 Quick Prescriptions for Mastering the Stress in Your Life.* Toronto, ON: QP Press.

Quit smoking support.com. (2011). *Have you ever wondered what's in a cigarette?* Retrieved from www.quitsmokingsupport.com/whatsinit.htm.

Selye, H. (1978). *The Stress of Life.* Colombus, OH: McGraw-Hill.

Smart Heart Living. (2010). *They say laughter is the best medicine.* Retrieved from www.smart-heart-living.com/laughter.html.

## Chapter 10. The Happiness Factor

A.A. Grapevine, Inc. (2001). *Alcoholics Anonymous 4th Ed.* New York City, NY: Alcoholics Anonymous World Services, Inc.

Kirshenbaum, M. (2003). *The Emotional Energy Factor: The Secrets High-energy People Use to Beat Emotional Fatigue.* New York, NY: Bantam Dell.

Nedd, K. (2009). *The Time to Be Happy Is Now.* Toronto, ON: QP Press.

Rubin, G. (2009). *The Happiness Project.* Toronto: Collins Canada.

Gordon, J. (2007). *The Energy Bus: 10 Rules to Fill Your Life, Work and Team with Positive Energy.* New Jersey: John Wiley & Sons, Inc.

Seligman, M (1990). *Learned Optimism: How to Change your Mind and Your Life.* New York, NY: Pocket Books.

## Chapter 11. The Kindness Experiment

Australian Kindness Movement. (1999, June). *Kindness and health.* Retrieved from www.kindness.com.au/kindness-and-health.html.

City of Richmond. (2005, April 12). *Richmond RCMO and city issue positive tickets.* Retrieved from www.richmond.ca/news/2005_city/tickets.htm.

Dossey, L. (1992). *Meaning and Medicine.* New York, NY: Bantam.

Lazare, A. (2010, December 10). *Go ahead, say you are sorry.* Retrieved from www.psychologytoday.com/articles/200909/go-ahead-say-youre-sorry.

Luks, A, & Payne, P. (2001). *The Healing Power of Doing Good.* Bloomington, IN : iUniverse.

Moreno, E. (2011). *The empowerment weekly.* Retrieved from www.empowermentweekly.com/2011/04/kindness-loving-heart-is-good-for-your.html.

Random Acts of Kindness Foundation. (2010). *Random acts of kindness.* Retrieved from www.randomactsofkindness.org.

Selkirk, D. (2009). *Catching kids being good.* Retrieved from www.shared-vision.com/svvisionaries/catching-kids-being-good.

The Healthy Living Site. (2011, January 07). *How acts of kindness benefit our health – plus 20 ways to pay-it-forward.* Retrieved from thehealthylivingsite.com/2011/01/how-acts-of-kindness-benefit-our-health-plus-20-ways-to-pay-it-forward.

## Chapter 12. The Passion Project

Cameron, J. (1992). *The Artist's Way: A Spiritual Path to Higher Creativity.* New York, NY: G.P. Putnam's Sons.

Golding, M. (1999). *Benjamin's Gift.* New York, NY: Grand Central Publishing.

McCoy, D.L. (1988). *Megatraits: 12 Traits of Successful People.* Plano, TX: Wordware Publishing, Inc.

Rasberry, S, & Selwyn, P. (1981). *Living Your Life Out Loud.* New York, NY: Pocket Books.

Whitworth, L, Kimsey-House, K, Kimsey-House, H, & Sandahl, P. (2009). *Co-Active Coaching.* Boston, MA: Nicholas Brealey Publishing.

# ABOUT THE AUTHOR

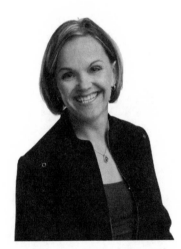

MICHELLE CEDERBERG is highly credentialed as a fitness and health professional holding a masters in kinesiology, a bachelors in psychology, and a specialization in exercise and health psychology. She is a certified exercise physiologist, and a certified life coach. She has over twenty years of practical experience working directly with clients in the fitness industry as a personal trainer and group exercise leader, and in daily life as a life coach and professional speaker.

About ten years ago Michelle went through a low patch where she was uninspired, low-energy, and unfulfilled in her work and personal life. She was a personal trainer who didn't value her own health, and as a professional speaker on life balance and stress management she felt like a phony because neither was working well in her life. The ideas in her book are part research and part personal experience from embracing a small-steps approach to get her life back on track. Her journey started with physical health as the foundation and built from there. She's lived most of what she writes about.

As a fifteen-year veteran in professional speaking and a certified speaking professional, Michelle has her finger on the pulse of the time, energy, and motivation challenges of her busy audience members, and was inspired to create her book as a tool to help them get and stay energized after her sessions are over. She speaks 12 months a year to diverse audiences across North America, sharing her expertise in a humorous, practical, and change-provoking way. Her weekly email messages and blog posts, as well as her hilarious Energy TV Youtube video segments, share more of Michelle's philosophy in her unique and entertaining style.

She lives in Calgary, Alberta, Canada with Ewan and their dog Lilly. Her website is www.worklifeenergy.com.

Sentient Publications, LLC publishes books on cultural creativity, experimental education, transformative spirituality, holistic health, new science, ecology, and other topics, approached from an integral viewpoint. Our authors are intensely interested in exploring the nature of life from fresh perspectives, addressing life's great questions, and fostering the full expression of the human potential. Sentient Publications' books arise from the spirit of inquiry and the richness of the inherent dialogue between writer and reader.

Our Culture Tools series is designed to give social catalyzers and cultural entrepreneurs the essential information, technology, and inspiration to forge a sustainable, creative, and compassionate world.

We are very interested in hearing from our readers. To direct suggestions or comments to us, or to be added to our mailing list, please contact:

SENTIENT PUBLICATIONS, LLC
1113 Spruce Street
Boulder, CO 80302
303-443-2188
contact@sentientpublications.com
www.sentientpublications.com